Data Presentation
and
Visual Literacy
in
Medicine and Science

Data Presentation
and
Visual Literacy
in
Medicine and Science

Doig Simmonds MAA

Formerly head of Medical Illustration at the Royal Postgraduate
Medical School, Hammersmith Hospital, London, UK

Linda Reynolds BSc MSc

Formerly Senior Research Fellow at the Royal College of Art; now
Visiting Lecturer at University of Reading, UK, and Freelance
Consultant in Information Design

Foreword by Dr Stephen Lock, Editor Emeritus of the
British Medical Journal

Illustrated by Doig Simmonds

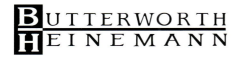
BUTTERWORTH
HEINEMANN

1994

Butterworth-Heinemann Ltd
Linacre House, Jordan Hill, Oxford OX2 8DP

ℛ A member of the Reed Elsevier group

Oxford London Boston
Munich New Delhi Singapore Sydney
Tokyo Toronto Wellington

First published 1994

British Library Cataloguing in Publication Data
A catalogue record for this book is available from the British Library

ISBN 0 7506 0982 6

Printed in Great Britain at the University Press, Cambridge

CONTENTS

FOREWORD

This book has two telling strengths. First, for a dinosaur who, pampered by a secretary all his professional life, suddenly finds himself on his own, the Apple Mac is a lifesaver. Hence I was delighted to see Simmonds and Reynolds laying such emphasis on it; to be sure, few PCs could be simpler, but they taught me a lot more about this marvellous machine.

Second, and more important, is their emphasis on the newer aspects of preparing graphics, for paradoxically here the computer is often the villain. As an editor and an attender at conferences, I have often been appalled at the abysmal quality of most illustrations for articles and slides for projection; the authors have been seduced by the possibilities of computer graphics programs. Simplicity and clarity are what consumers need, and Simmonds and Reynolds are adept at explaining how to achieve both.

Nevertheless the real nugget of this book is the chapter on preparing posters, those low-ranking consolation prizes in professional esteem (for, just as some journals sweeten the pill of rejecting an article by offering the author a Letter to the Editor, so do some conference organisers divert meretricious rubbish into posters). But many third-rate posters also originate in good quality science — though the results are the same: hundreds of words in small print, complex tables, and strings of references, impelling the reader to turn to the next poster, which is invariably just as bad. For a few years I judged 450 posters at my old teaching hospital's annual postgraduate meeting. It took less than an hour, I found, to recognise the four or five that had real merit. The authors had realised that, like lectures and talks, posters are totally different from formal written articles: a form of show business, they need catchy readable titles, bright graphics, few words, and a clear message — with the science presented in a detailed handout.

'Think, work, publish', said the great Michael Farraday — a sentiment echoed in our own times by the physicist-philosopher John Ziman: 'The object of science is publication'. Both statements emphasise that failure to publish (which includes presentations and posters at conferences) is a reflection of poor ethical standards. To take the idea further, I would suggest that indifference to doing things correctly is almost as heinous. After this book there can be no excuse for such boorishness.

STEPHEN LOCK
Editor BMJ 1975-91

ACKNOWLEDGEMENTS

The authors wish to thank the members of staff of the Royal Post-graduate Medical School and Hammersmith Hospital for sharing in our efforts to establish standards of visual literacy and for helping in so many ways to support the experiences covered in this book. We are also grateful to the School for permission to use some of the illustrative work created while Doig Simmonds was employed there.

To Martinus Nijhoff and Kluwer Academic Publishers we also owe thanks for returning the copyright of our previous books, first published by them: *Presentation of Data in Science* and *Computer Presentation of Data in Science.*

Frank Sketch of PCSS Consultants has always been an invaluable aid and support whenever we needed advice on any matters concerning computers, both IBM and Macintosh.

We are grateful to Maeve O'Connor, secretary to the European Association of Science Editors, for editorial checking and suggestions, and in particular to Stephen Lock, Editor Emeritus of the British Medical Journal, for his useful comments and for agreeing to write the foreword.

Louise Perks and Jane Fallows, formerly on the medical illustration staff at RPMS, have been very supportive colleagues. We are particularly grateful to Louise Perks for the work she did several years ago in teaching the medical staff how to draw graphs and charts efficiently; some of our examples are based on her work.

We have also drawn from our own previously published work in The Electronic Author, a publication of the Society of Authors, and in JAMM, the Journal of the Institute of Medical Illustration. We have also drawn from 'Charts and Graphs', edited by Doig Simmonds and produced for the former Institute of Medical and Biological Illustration.

This book is entirely the responsibility of the authors, who wrote it, illustrated it, designed it from cover to cover and typeset it. Any errors are our responsibility and are very much regretted.

INTRODUCTION

1

Who is this book for and what is it about? Why is it needed? The desktop publishing revolution and the new freedom this has provided, plus the new pitfalls. 'Publish or Perish' — the pressure of competition. Why are papers often rejected? The importance of design principles and of matching form and function. Why choose an Apple Macintosh computer? The compatibility of programs and data, both within the chosen system and with 'foreign' data. Changes in the workplace environment.

Who is this book for?

This book is for all those who are new to the business of using computer technology in the design and production of scientific information, whether it be in the form of a handout, a contribution to a journal, a commercially printed publication, a slide or overhead transparency, or a poster presentation at a scientific meeting.

Now that we have banished the specialists from the ranks of our service departments and have to do everything ourselves, we need to obtain some of those specialist skills. Anyone who buys a computer can, in effect, become a writer, designer, typographer, artist, and desktop publisher overnight, but many of us then find that we lack the knowledge to produce professional results. The people who suffer are the 'consumers' of the information — the readers of reports and journals, and the lecture audiences — who have to face those overcrowded tables and unreadable slides, now so beautifully produced!

What is this book about?

A literate person is one who has learned the rules of reading, writing and comprehension. We have learned to take these rules

Visual literacy

for granted. Poets and novelists may extend and develop the rules from time to time but, for most of us, the basics are all we need to communicate our ideas. This book sets out to provide some of the fundamental rules for good communication.

There is evidence to suggest that the way we 'read' pictures and type is indeed subject to certain basic 'laws' of perception, and there are many well-established principles in graphic design that are in keeping with these laws. We believe that it is usually counter-productive to ignore design principles that have been well tested over time and whose value in many cases has been confirmed by research. We seek to signpost these principles throughout the book, and to offer you guidelines for structured thought about design so that you can establish a style of your own to suit your method of working and your circumstances.

Computer literacy There are many distinct advantages to using computer technology. Digital methods mean that you can now forget about pens, inks, pencils, erasers, compasses, paste, tape, spray-glue, rub-down lettering, and all the rest of the physical junk that sticks to your elbows, gets borrowed by someone or is eaten by the dog just when you need it. Massive amounts of data can be stored in compact form, making them easy to transport and easy to manipulate. Scanning technology has reached the point where existing documents can be incorporated into new ones without the need for retyping data. Drawings and photographs can be manipulated in a variety of ways. Once data are digitized, they can be combined with other data in an infinite variety of ways. All the advantages are, however, balanced by an impressive array of pitfalls for the unwary. We also provide information about operator working comfort and health, computer viruses and security from 'hackers', and give advice that may prevent disasters such as disc crashes and loss of data.

Why is this book needed?

The so-called 'desktop publishing revolution', using computer technology and laserprinters, has given rise to a massive amount of well-printed but badly-designed material, produced amazingly fast and very cheaply. Two examples of this are the preparation of lecture slides and of papers for publication.

Illegible lecture slides We all look with wonder at what the Professor has been able to produce in the lunch hour — twenty five slides in almost as many minutes — but can you read them? He has used a wonderful decorative typeface called Chancery Zapf and has given it all sorts of

Chancery Zapf with Outline and Shadow effects

'enhancements'. This might be acceptable on a visiting card but certainly cannot be read at the back of the lecture hall. The Professor has decided to have blue diazo slides. By using a new, instant, do-it-yourself slide-maker he has been able to produce these *five minutes* before his lecture. (Will wonders never cease?) His students decide that they will skip his lectures in future; this is the *n*th time that they have had to suffer not only illegible slides but a different typeface on each occasion as well. Eventually the Professor tires of his new toy and so hands it over to his secretary, telling her, 'It's so terribly easy to use'. To her amazement, it is. She *loves* the underline style — it's automatic! She uses it whenever she likes, which is often. The Professor still wonders why students don't turn up for lectures.

Underlining interferes with the lower parts of the lettering

It has been said that 'research unpublished has not been done', but competition to get into print, caused by the current dictum of 'publish or perish' existing in so many institutions of higher education and research, often results in hasty work. This not only affects the quality of research but also the quality of the presented material.

__The rejection of papers__

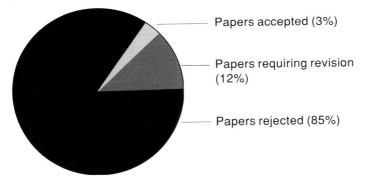

Papers accepted (3%)

Papers requiring revision (12%)

Papers rejected (85%)

The pie-chart shows the acceptance rate for scientific papers submitted to learned journals. These figures are common to many of the major scientific journals. It is a buyer's market. Only about 3% of papers submitted for publication are accepted with no revision needed. Some 12% will require some revision and a massive 85% are rejected. We are indebted to Dr Stephen Lock, Editor Emeritus of the British Medical Journal, for this information and for giving us the following common reasons for rejection:

- *Material unsuitable for the journal in question.* This means that the author has not examined the current fashion in subject matter of the particular journal.

- *Papers badly written, with poor use of language.* There are many books to help the author here (see under 'Further reading').

- *Inadequate scientific basis for the work.* Help can usually be had from others in the field.

- *Poor statistics.* Again, help is needed from specialists, and there are many useful books available.

- *Confusing illustrations.* Help is needed with drawings and design techniques. It is not so easy to get advice on these matters, and this is where we expect our book to fill a gap.

REJECTED   ACCEPTED

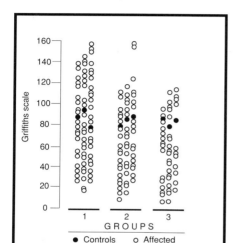 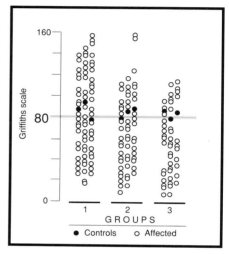

The 'mean' line at 80 was missing when the graph was first submitted. This simple omission caused a delay of several months in publication

Design principles

The kinds of difficulties described above result from a lack of knowledge of basic design principles and failure to take into account the design constraints imposed by different media.

In spite of the fact that conventional typesetting has been replaced with electronic systems, the traditions of design established for solid type still hold true. Digital type, however, is free of the constraints imposed by solid letterforms. We can close up, expand, stretch and shrink lettering, or even bubble it as if it were chewing gum. But if we want our work to convey information effectively as well as look attractive, the old design principles must not be ignored.

Length of line, line spacing, the size of type for a given reading distance and the basic forms of the letters themselves cannot be varied very much without causing visual chaos. Wordprocessing and electronic page make-up have given all of us unlimited freedom to create such chaos. If, however, we choose to follow some of the obvious and sensible signposts established by designers in the past, we can enjoy our new-found freedom and at the same time produce results that are attractive, easy to read, created at short notice and infinitely editable.

The design of tables is one of the commonest problems facing those new to wordprocessing on a computer, and yet there is nothing easier to master. Unlike the typewriter, the computer gives complete control over tabulation. Numerals or texts can be aligned in four different ways and the type size can be selected to suit the content of the table and the medium in which it will be shown.

The use of colour is also discussed. In general it is commonly misused merely as a decorative enhancement. There has to be a sensible justification for its use and the main one is that colour can play a vital role in coding information.

Form and function

The possibilities and limitations of the presentation medium involved must also be taken into account. Form and function have to be related. A chair that does not conform to the shape of the human body is not comfortable to sit on. Similarly, when we are presenting information of any kind to other people we should design it to perform the specific function we intend. This therefore implies that data designed for presentation in one form are not likely to be suitable for presentation in another. Material designed for a 35mm slide will not be suitable for an overhead projector transparency nor for electronic projection systems.The document you have designed for a student handout is unlikely to be accepted for publication in a scientific journal. We give design guidelines for each of these different kinds of presentation.

Apple Macintosh and Power PC

It will soon become obvious, if you get beyond this introduction, that most of what we discuss in this book has been based on the use of Apple Macintosh computers and software, now also incorporated into the Power PC. The reason for preferring this environment is that both computers use a 'graphic' interface between the machine and the user to produce effects, rather than a complex 'formula' based language. This graphic basis means that you get a more accurate impression on the screen of what the outcome of your work will be. The IBM and its clones are trying to catch up in this respect but they are still disadvantaged by older, formula-based technology and its resulting cumbersome graphics. However, 'Windows' technology, with its smarter graphics borrowed from the Macintosh, is now established in the IBM environment.

The Macintosh and Power PC computers also offer additional features not found in other technology. The most important of these is the fact that *all* the programs use the *same* operating system and this is installed just once. This operating system contains all the fonts, symbols and other paraphernalia that you may want to use and they are available for any other program. For example, the 'Find' facility is available to find lost files whatever program is currently in use. There is a 'magic' Scrapbook which acts as a convenient store for any images, either drawings or texts, which you may wish to repeat, and they don't dissolve when you switch the machine off but remain for use permanently. You may, for example, have designed an equation which you want to store and use over and over again. The Macintosh will store this image in its Scrapbook for your use at any time, for use by all programs. The IBM and clones cannot do this yet. The Power PC has the greatest advantage of all, and that is that it can run any IBM 'Windows' program *as well as* Macintosh programs, simultaneously. Fortunately many of the older Macintosh machines can be upgraded to Power PCs. The unfortunate IBM owner cannot yet do this. IBM, Motorola and Apple have co-operated to make the Power PC and this is the next generation of computers.

All Apple/ Power PC programs are compatible one with another, and provided your system is suitably upgraded and 'memory' is sufficient, you can switch instantly between them. Because of the relative simplicity of the Macintosh operating system, most of the manuals are short and easy to understand. The majority are also laid out in a uniform manner. Tutorials are usually provided and these are an excellent way of learning the basics of any new program. In a later chapter we recommend a few basic programs for those starting out in this technology.

The workplace

Developments in information technology are altering attitudes towards work. Fax machines, scanners and modems now allow us to exchange data down the telephone line and so give us the freedom to work at home or in small and more comfortable offices. Geography is no longer important, and the way people are employed will change as institutions and individuals respond to computer technology.

CHOOSING YOUR COMPUTER SYSTEM AND SOFTWARE

2

Shopping around is vital, not just for price but also for the reliability and commercial reputation of suppliers. Have you decided what you want to use a computer for? Will it be easy to learn? Is there an ideal configuration for your needs? How much memory is necessary? What output devices (printers for paper and for slides) are needed? What should I look for when I buy software? Compatibility: can I use data produced by other computers?

Finding out what's available

The over-abundance of computer hardware, software, journals and jargon that exists in so many industrialised countries can be very confusing to the beginner.

You have to start somewhere. Begin by deciding exactly what you want a computer for. Is it just to make the production of scientific papers easier? Are you interested in writing books that will require footnotes and glossaries? Or are you more interested in some sort of analytical system that will help you in medical diagnosis, patient care or drug therapy? Do you want to manage a complex database, perform calculations, draw graphs showing the results and link these to a publication? Are you keen to produce overhead transparencies, good slides and plenty of publication-quality illustrations? Do you perhaps need to combine several of these requirements — is there a 'do it all' kind of software? Are you in a situation where you may wish to expand your work to embrace more complex tasks in the future, perhaps going from simple wordprocessing to publishing patient information booklets involving photographs and drawings?

Decisions, decisions!

The most important rule to observe when choosing a system is to look before you leap, and the best advice we can give is to echo what has already been said by James Felici and Ted Nace in their excellent book, 'Desktop Publishing Skills':

Learn from others

"Really useful guidance can *only be had from other users* [our italics] of the system you are considering — and not just any users, but those who have applied the system to documents similar to yours. Don't buy a system until you have talked to such users. If you can't find any, ask your vendor for the names of two or three."

It is useful to read a selection of computer journals, go to computer exhibitions, and learn the jargon. Jargon is important because it is inescapable. It is also a short-cut that helps to avoid lengthy description. The problem with jargon is that it is bandied about by vendors in such a manner as to confuse the novice, so let the novice learn and also be aware of the pitfalls of jargon. A term like WYSIWYG — 'What You See Is What You Get' — isn't a precisely true statement. This term suggests that what you see on the screen is what you are going to get as the final product. However, the screen version of an image can only be an approximate representation of the final printed version because of the differences that exist between resolution on a computer screen (72 dots per inch) and the resolution of printers (commonly from 300 dots per inch upwards).

The vital statistics of computers

In March 1994 a consortium of Apple, IBM and Motorola launched a new computer called the 'Power PC'. Power PCs use RISC co-processor technology rather than the former CISC technology, the latter now being doomed to die a natural death. Understanding the jargon is not vital to the new purchaser, but what is vital is that he or she appreciates a few simple points. First, the Power PC offers the purchaser the speed and versatility formerly associated with much more expensive computers, but at 'high-street affordability'. The purchasing choice for a newcomer is to buy either a Power PC or a secondhand Apple Macintosh which can be upgraded to the Power PC. The most important advantage of the Power PC is that it can run programs designed for either MS-DOS Windows or Macintosh environments. The Power PC is rated as operating between two and five times faster than any other PC or Macintosh. This machine now dissolves the former dichotomy between the IBM MS-DOS 'formula-driven' environments and the Macintosh 'QuickDraw' environment, which often led to battles between the advocates of each system. The Power PC will accept discs formatted for either MS-DOS or Macintosh.

New software now being developed will make multi-tasking much easier as the trend is towards integrated programs which provide many functions including writing, drawing, statistics and communication. This kind of flexibility will allow you to be more professional and more efficient.

Memory — computers need a lot!

All computers have some sort of resident memory, and the size of *RAM and ROM* this memory will determine what you can and can't do with your system. The memory consists of two separate parts, the read-only memory (ROM) and the random access memory (RAM). The ROM is essential for the operation of programs, remembering what has to be sent to the printing device, and general computer housekeeping. The RAM is the working space required for handling programs and data. You must make sure that your computer has enough RAM to cope with your particular demands. For our purposes, memory is measured in megabytes and kilobytes. One megabyte (MB) is equal to 1000 kilobytes (K).

The more sophisticated the program and the more it is able to do *How much RAM?* for you, the larger the size of the RAM needed for efficient operation. For example, the minimum RAM requirement for using System 7 on the Macintosh is two megabytes, but if you include multi-functional programs such as may be required for general scientific work, then you will need much more. Four megabytes is an acceptable minimum. The less the RAM memory the less likely you are to be able to graduate to more complex activities.

The Power PC requires sixteen megabytes of RAM if you want to work with IBM Windows, otherwise you can get by with eight megabytes. Not having enough RAM is a common complaint. Most people soon reach the point of saying: 'If only I had bought a machine with more memory then I could have used a more sophisticated program and got my work done more efficiently'. We recommend eight megabytes as a minimum. Make sure you buy a kit which is capable of easy expansion. It is worth asking whether upgrading the RAM and ROM is simply a matter of plugging in new units, or whether the software needs to be reconfigured.

The memory requirements of a number of programs are mentioned later to help you in choosing your hardware. You must also have sufficient free memory available not only to run the program but also to temporarily store your current work.

Another vital question, and one that is often neglected, is: What do you expect as the final printout? Do you want a book-quality product? Do you want near-perfect graphics such as may be needed by those producing audiovisual teaching materials? Or are you simply content with a decently produced page of text that will be printed later by other means? If you want top quality output, then you must choose a computer and software that will enable you to link up with an imagesetter. If quality is not that important, you will probably be content with a setup that outputs to an inkjet printer or personal laserprinter. But do ask yourself whether your requirements are ever likely to change. Plan for growth.

User friendliness   User-friendliness is another important factor to consider. The Apple Macintosh was designed and developed as 'The computer for the rest of us'. As a graphics-driven machine it uses pictures (icons) to tell us what things are, a manually operated pointer to drive around the screen (mouse), and a useful on-screen helpline with pull-down menus in case we get lost and need advice while in the middle of a job. Many of these built-in 'help' facilities are so good that the manuals become redundant.

Well-thought-out manuals   The design and layout of instruction manuals are often useful indicators as to whether a system is easy to use or complex and difficult. Top-level products provide manuals which are laid out in a manner that makes repeated reference easy. They are usually spiral-bound so that they open flat, and are not too large. This means that the open manual can be placed within easy reach for reference while operating the computer. The typeface chosen is clear and the text is set out in columns rather than right across the page. A good manual usually has one clear heading to each page and commonly deals with only one subject or problem per page or column. There is often plenty of space in the margins, with shoulder headings for easy selection of subject matter. Margin space is very useful if you need to make your own comments and notes. The whole design is such that repeated glances can be made comfortably and easily without any tendency to lose your place. Using a low-quality manual is more like trying to find your train from a railway timetable or a telephone number in a directory. A casual glance to look for a reminder about a specific technique is often impossible with badly designed manuals.

If you have reached the point where something takes your fancy, are you sure that it is robust and rugged in design? Many low-cost popular 'home' computers are not rugged and sometimes servicing is non-existent. So find out who are the vendors in your area and whether they have a good reputation. Is there a reliable backup service for the computer you're thinking about? As far as service is concerned, the vendor will always tell you how good it is, so try to get an independent opinion.

Hardware — the computer

Computers can either be supplied as one unit or in modular form. The unit will consist of a box containing the electronics and the hard disc, and above this a screen for viewing the image. If, later on, you find that you need a bigger screen, you will have to buy a whole new machine. It is better to purchase the computer and screen separately so that each can be upgraded or exchanged for better models independently.

The computer itself comes with at least one high density 3.5 inch floppy disc drive as well as a choice of internal hard drives. The floppy disc drive will accept 'high density' as well as 'double density' discs. Double density discs can store a nominal 800 kilobytes of information. High density discs have the letters 'HD' in the top right corner and an open slot in the bottom right corner. These discs can store up to 1400 kilobytes (nominal) of data. Both HD and DD discs can be made compatible with, and formatted for, MS-DOS machines. This is unique to the Macintosh and Power PC which are the machines of choice in our opinion. Nearly all Macintosh word-processing software will import or export IBM-generated data. The computer must have output ports at the back for peripheral devices such as the printer, or for any add-on you may want later such as an extra hard drive or a modem.

Label: HD

Extra hole in corner

The monitor (viewing screen)

An important factor to consider when choosing a monitor is the size. Most users would like to see at least the top half of the paper they are working on, or preferably the whole sheet. Screen sizes are measured across the screen diagonally. This means that a 14-inch (35cm) monitor is the minimum requirement. A 19-inch (48cm) diagonal will allow you to display two A4 sheets of paper arranged vertically side by side. There are A4 monitors that will rotate so that the screen view is either portrait (long axis vertical) or landscape (long axis horizontal). The latter view is particularly useful for large spreadsheets. If money is tight and you can't afford what you want, then take heart from the fact that all Macintosh programs allow you to enlarge your view of the window (zoom in) or reduce it (zoom out).

Is a colour monitor important? Colour becomes necessary if you are producing colour slides and want to see exactly what is going on. It is also helpful as a highlighter on the screen. For example, most wordprocessing and page make-up programs have guidelines and rulers which, when displayed in colour, are helpful. We would advise buying a colour monitor if you can afford it. It has to be remembered that colour uses up more RAM, but a colour monitor can also be operated in black-and-white mode which saves a lot of memory.

The keyboard — standard and extended

Macintosh computer keyboards are customisable. It may be desirable to change the keyboard layout if you have keyboard operators who speak languages other than that for which the computer was originally purchased. The QWERTY keyboard does not exist in France for example. The Macintosh (and IBM) keyboards can temporarily or permanently be restyled to suit a very large selection of world languages using a 'localising' software. The extended keyboard is a must for the scientist who is going to deal a lot with numbers. The standard keyboard is extended to include a section to the right with duplicate numeric and math function keys so that they are much quicker to use. There are versions for lefthanded users too.

Peripherals — extra hard drives, scanners, modems

Removable hard discs Storage of data soon becomes a problem. The hard disc within the machine will very quickly get cluttered up if you do not have storage elsewhere. Keeping work permanently within the computer is a very bad idea. What if there is a disc crash? All your work can be destroyed for ever. It is essential to have storage elsewhere. High density floppy discs can store only a nominal 1400K each, so it makes sense to have a removable hard drive or an optical drive as peripheral storage if you have large amounts of data to deal with. A removable hard drive such as the SyQuest™ can use discs of 44-megabyte or 88-megabyte capacity. The 3.5 inch re-writable optical discs can store 128 megabytes **Re-writable optical discs** of data. Optical discs are the safest of all because the data are not prone to damage by dust, heat, damp or magnetism; the other discs mentioned *are* sensitive to these factors.

Scanners Scanners become important if you want to import and digitise hardcopy in the form of photographs, drawings or typed/printed texts. There are cylinder scanners, flatbed scanners and hand-held roller scanners. The latter are slightly cheaper than flatbed scanners.

Modems Modems are used for communication. They use the normal telephone line and can be very useful if you need to be constantly in touch with others. However, they may occupy your machine time at inconvenient moments unless you have a separate computer dedicated to this function. They can also be dangerous as a source of unwelcome foreign data such as viruses or junk mail.

The mouse or the stylus

These are tools for manipulating the image on screen. A mouse is supplied as part of the computer. It takes some people time to get used to it. It's like trying to draw with a bar of soap! Styluses on the other hand have to be purchased and are relatively expensive. They feel like a normal pen. The best are pressure sensitive and have no wires to get in the way. However, a mouse is often more accurate when it comes to placing objects at precise points on the screen.

Printers for paper

Dot matrix printers have a single print head consisting of a series of pins that strike the paper in various configurations to form the characters. These printers do not produce results of publishable quality and are not worth considering.   ***Dot matrix printers***

Inkjet printers such as the StyleWriter™ fire tiny jets of ink onto the paper. The image produced is very good quality, having a resolution of 300 dots per inch or more, and is perfectly suitable for publication. The method is slower than laserprinting, however, and the ink is not stable under extreme conditions such as high humidity or excessive light. Accidentally wetting the paper will cause the image to smudge. Graphics and lettering of any size are possible within the limits of the paper available.   ***Inkjet printers***

Laserprinters have a standard minimum resolution of 300dpi, but can go up to 600 or even 1200dpi. Laserprinting is 'permanent' in the sense that, because the image is made of carbon dust and is fused to the paper by heat, it is not liable to damage from excesses of heat or humidity.   ***Laserprinters***

Imagesetters such as the Linotron™ have image resolutions from 1270dpi to 2540dpi. These machines produce film for litho printing, or high quality photographic bromide prints for camera-ready work. They are priced well beyond the means of most readers of this book, but they can operate directly from the same humble 3.5-inch disk that you use in your computer.   ***Imagesetters***

Printers for 35mm slide or OHP

There are printers designed to produce transparencies straight from disc. Work has to be formatted to 35mm or OHP requirements and we mention two good programs to do this job: Aldus Persuasion 2™ and Microsoft PowerPoint 3™. Expensive printers are needed to produce slides of acceptable quality and it is best to use a specialist bureau service. Low-cost, do-it-yourself printers such as those using the Polaroid system are inclined to produce poor quality results.

Printers and fonts

The lettering that printing machines of all kinds use is divided up into families called 'fonts'. These all have names, such as 'Times Roman™', 'Helvetica™' and so on. But many of these names are protected by copyright law, so something that may be based on

Times Roman™ could be slightly altered and called 'TimRom' or even 'New York'. You do have to know your way around fonts in order to get your work to look the way you want it to, or to comply with a publisher's specifications.

We will deal with fonts in greater detail in Chapter 4, but for now it is enough to know that there is an important difference between fonts used by the printing device and fonts used on your monitor screen. Laserprinters and imagesetters use fonts which emulate the typefaces traditionally used in book publishing and advertising. As well as screen versions of these fonts, there are screen fonts (such as Geneva on the Macintosh) that have been specially designed for clarity on the screen, but for which there are no printer equivalents. If you attempt to print one of these screen fonts, the printer will either substitute an alternative font or provide an unsatisfactory bitmapped image. This can cause a heavy increase in printing time, and in the case of 35mm slide printers may even stop output altogether.

General software for the scientist

What follows is advice based not only on our own experience but also on the opinion of scientists who use the software mentioned to produce work for publication or teaching. We discuss software for wordprocessing, statistics, equations, drawings, databases and spreadsheets. We will mainly consider software suitable at entry level but we will also mention software that you may want to move on to for more professional results. We have not attempted to give a comprehensive list of features for each program mentioned below, but have listed those which we think you should examine when you ask around.

The majority of the Macintosh/Power PC programs mentioned are supported by well-designed manuals with on-screen 'help' facilities which are mini-versions of the manual. In many cases an animated on-screen video training section is included on the software disc, which takes you through the main features of the program. A common feature in all Macintosh programs is the ability to enlarge or reduce the view. The reduced view allows you to see the entire layout of a page at a glance and the enlarged view allows you to smarten up the details.

A growing number of programs try to do everything you want, but the chances are that you will have to purchase more than one program to function efficiently. Separately, wordprocessing programs process words and are limited in their design features. Page make-up programs are principally design tools for creating complete documents, such as books. Although they may include limited drawing facilities, such as the ability to surround text with ovals, boxes or toned backgrounds, they are not true drawing programs. Statistical programs are good at processing numbers (number crunching) but are limited in their drawing ability, and so it goes on. There are some very good drawing programs that have limited wordprocessing facilities. Let us emphasise once again the importance of finding out what other people in your field are doing and what computers and programs they are using. All of the wordprocessing programs mentioned here have good dictionaries, spell-checkers, a thesaurus and the essential translators for importing IBM PC documents and some other 'foreign' formats. Numbers in brackets are the recommended RAM requirements (in kilobytes) needed to operate the program.

ClarisWorks II™ (950K)

ClarisWorks™ is a 'do-it-all' program which combines word- **Do-it-all** processing (based on MacWrite™), database (based on **programs** FileMaker™), spreadsheet with statistics (based on Resolve™), graphics (based on MacDraw™) and communications software, all for less than £100 (UK educational price in April 1993). This program is fantastic value. The manual is good, there is on-screen help, and there is a training video which covers all sections of this excellent program. We know of postgraduate students who have produced entire theses using the wordprocessing, spreadsheet and graphics facilities of ClarisWorks™. The spreadsheet will allow you to produce graphs, but unfortunately it lacks the ability to automatically introduce standard error bars. These can be added by plotting stacked bars then adjusting these in the drawing mode (see page 108).

There are several very useful features in ClarisWorks™. The graphic toolbox can be called up and used in any of the other sections of the program, so lines, boxes, etc. can be added even in wordprocessing or spreadsheet mode. In drawing mode, text boxes can be designed so that text flows automatically between them. This makes the design of posters for scientific meetings particularly easy. However, the rotation of text is limited to 90° increments only. Arrows can be customised to suit almost any requirement, and drawings can be dimensioned automatically.

The wordprocessing mode has automatic footnote numbering which will rearrange the footnotes should you change the numbers. The mailmerge feature makes standard letters easy. Tables are particularly well dealt with as you can import a spreadsheet window into a wordprocessed document and thus control the alignment and spacing of numbers without recourse to setting tabs. Numbers can then be edited within fields without upsetting the line of text. Search and replace facilities are very thorough and apply to all modes. Pages can be designed to have up to nine columns for text. This feature makes it easy to produce newsletters or organise student handouts.

The spreadsheet mode provides eight function categories: Business & Financial, Date & Time, Information, Logical, Numeric, Statistical, Text, and finally, Trigonometric.

MacWrite Pro™ (1025K)

This is now one of the premier wordprocessing programs for the Macintosh. It enables the user to produce page layout work that formerly could be done only in very expensive programs such as PageMaker™ or QuarkExpress™. MacWrite Pro™ does this by allowing you to create text or table frames wherever you want on the page. You can 'link' them or not as you please. When linked, text flows from one frame to the next.

WriteNow 3™ (490K)

Wordprocessing only

An exceptionally fast and very easy to use wordprocessing program with all the important basic facilities such as mailmerge, dictionaries, thesaurus, etc..

CricketGraph III™ (1200K)

Graphing program

This is a good general statistical program that deals very efficiently with converting spreadsheet data into graphs of all the most commonly used kinds. CricketGraph™ copes very efficiently with standard error bars in a variety of formats. There are 23 plot symbols to choose from, as well as a plot symbol of 'none' should you wish to have continuous lines plotted through invisible points. The graph types available are: scatter, line, bar, column, stacked bar, stacked column, area, pie, polar and quality control. Curve-fitting is based on: linear, power, logarithmic, exponential, polynomial and interpolation. The equations used can be displayed or not as you wish. Graphic enhancements of graphs, such as space between bars, the colour or tone of each bar and the way axes are drawn, are all user-definable. Graphs can be overlaid, i.e. one kind over another. Several windows can be opened at the same time so that graphs can be compared.

CricketGraph™ is not the only statistical/graphing package available but it is a sound and easy to use program, tried and tested by many scientists.

MacDraw II™ (581K), MacDraw Pro™ (2000K) and MacDraft III™ (1500K)

Drawing programs

These are all drawing programs which deal very effectively with most of the needs of the scientist who wishes to produce diagrams. Wordprocessing facilities are also included so that it becomes possible to produce good-looking layouts by creating 'text blocks'. This is something that many wordprocessors cannot do because of the way the text has to proceed from line to line in sequence. Trying to produce a table in a wordprocessing program can sometimes pose a problem because of this (except for MacWrite Pro™ and Microsoft Word 5.1™). It is often easier to create a table in a 'draw' program or as an implanted spreadsheet. In the latter case, each column is a separate entity. MacDraft™ has two advantages that the others do not have. Firstly, it can calculate the area of any enclosed shape. This may be a useful feature for comparing cell sizes for example (see page 103). Secondly, MacDraft™ can draw arcs and circle segments in a variety of ways which give you full control over them; this is perfect for genome construction (see page 100). All three programs can rotate objects, including text, in 1–360° increments.

All of the drawing programs mentioned above can be used to create 35mm slides or overhead transparencies. It is therefore not necessary to purchase the dedicated programs mentioned below unless you produce a lot of slides.

MacPaint II™ (512K)

MacPaint is very useful for including little sketch-like drawings into work. Everything is 'bit-mapped', i.e. rather rough looking, but a lot of charming cartoon work has been done with this cheap and successful program. It is a 'fun' program with all sorts of artists' tools like paint brushes and an airbrush. However, a more powerful program such as IntelliDraw™ costs about the same.

MathType III™ (512K)

This program is a must for those who need to design complex equations. It works by using an infinitely expanding matrix system. Each matrix can be linked to others and can be customised to contain a variety of text/symbol styles. Brackets expand with increases in the enclosed matrices. *Equations*

Persuasion 2™ (1500K)

This is a fairly complex slide-making program based on word-processed input. Slides are automatically produced from an outline text. There are many pre-formed designs to use for slides. *35mm slides*

PowerPoint 3™ (1500K)

A simpler program which does a good job and is easier to learn than Persuasion™. Imported work isn't quite so easy to change.

OmniPage Professional™ (3700K)

OCR The best of several OCR (Optical Character Recognition) programs that convert scanned texts into digital (computer-usable) type without the need to re-key the work. This program cannot be used without a scanner.

Purchasing

We cannot give accurate figures for costing out your project. There are two avenues to explore. Firstly, if you are eligible for educational discounts these are very attractive. Secondly, try the many mail order houses. They may offer attractive prices based on those found in the country of origin. But be careful about them. The operating system for the computer may be unsuitable for or even incompatible with software designed for sale in your country. Standard page sizes in the USA are not the same as those in the rest of the world. Dictionaries and standard spellings vary, particularly between US English and UK English. Some pirated software may be available from countries that are not party to international agreements on copyright protection. Not only is it illegal to use such software but it may introduce viruses or be incomplete. Be careful about wonderful offers for hardware which include software as a bundled item. It may be a demonstration version only and may lack the ability to print. Always ask whether bundled software is a full version and whether it is the latest version.

'Bargain' software may be a false economy

Do not become a copyright thief Purchase your software. Do not be tempted to 'borrow' programs from others. Although it may seem a reasonable idea to try someone else's program before you embark on an expensive purchase, it is a breach of the copyright laws. It is in any case highly advantageous to be registered as the legitimate owner because this often entitles you to inexpensive or free upgrades. Software vendors may not always keep you posted when an upgrade is available. You must check on this by reading the relevant trade journals. It is important to upgrade whenever you can and within the time limit advertised. The improvements are usually worthwhile, and sometimes a virtually new program is offered for a fraction of the full purchase price.

Training

External training courses may not be necessary if you follow the tutorials that come with your machine and software in a patient and dedicated manner. Training courses in the commercial sector are numerous but expensive and often well beyond the pocket of the scientist. In any case, courses for those working in science subjects often have to be specifically designed for very particular needs. To find out what's available, it's well worth joining a user group or club devoted to your particular kind of work. You may then be eligible for certain low-cost training programmes. Alternatively, you may be able to find something suitable by a direct approach to your own vendor, local university or technical college, or through advertisements in the journals that deal with your system. Before you embark on a training course, you should familiarise yourself with the basics of your computer. Getting 'stuck in' and starting to teach yourself is by far the best way to begin. The experience of others is more likely to come in useful later, or when you want some specialist information that isn't in the manual.

What follows are our recommendations as to the minimum equipment needed by the scientist about to enter the world of computer-originated work.

Starter pack

Hardware

- Macintosh LC III: 4MB RAM, 80MB internal hard disc. Upgradable to 8MB RAM, 160MB hard disc, or larger if required. (Mouse is included.)
- Extended keyboard (includes numeric keypad) instead of the standard keyboard.
- 14-inch Apple colour monitor
- Apple StyleWriter™ printer.

Software

- ClarisWorks II™, MathType™ and CricketGraph III™ programs.
- Pack of ten high density 3.5-inch floppy discs for data storage.

The approximate 1993 education cost of the above: £1,500, including VAT.

To be added later

Hardware

- Memory upgrade cards.
- Optical, re-writable 128MB hard drive for data storage.
- Apple scanner.

Software

- OmniPage Professional™, PageMaker 5™, PhotoShop 2.5™. The choice of programs will depend on the work you do.

The approximate 1993 education cost of the additions above: £2,500, including VAT.

Memory needed for System 7 and some popular programs

System 7™	2000K minimum. Can easily become 20,000K with fonts and dictionaries!
CricketGraph III™	1200K. Graphs, including standard errors
ClarisWorks II™	950K. An integrated package containing five programs. Graphing does not include standard errors
MacDraft III™	1500K. Can be used to create 35mm slide and OHP presentations. Has the best drawing tools
MacDraw II™	900K. Can be used to create 35mm slide and OHP presentations
MacDraw Pro™	2000K. Can be used to create 35mm slide and OHP presentations
MathType III™	512K. Mathematics and equations program (includes a special font)
MacPaint II™	512K. Bitmapped freehand drawing and painting program
Persuasion 2™	1500K. 35mm slide and OHP presentation package
PowerPoint 3™	1500K. 35mm slide and OHP presentation package — memory can be reduced, see below
OmniPage Prof.™	3700K. OCR software, needs a scanner

Memory needed by more complex programs

These are listed to show you what not to buy when you start out. Buy them when you get to the professional stage — and when you can afford to!

Word 5.0™	1024K. A complex program, but useful for PC translation; MathType™ built in. Graphing does not include standard errors
Illustrator 5.0™	4700K. Professional drawing program with graphing facility (no standard errors)
FreeHand 4.0™	4000K. Professional drawing program. No graphing facility

PhotoShop 2.5™	5120K. Photographic manipulation and art-work program
PageMaker 5.0™	2750K. Professional typesetting and page make-up program, marvellous for book publication

The memory requirement stated is that recommended to operate the program, but the package will usually contain other items such as tutorials, samples, dictionaries etc.. These will obviously occupy even more memory space on your hard disc.

Recommended journals

MacUser
Charwood House
Marsh Road
Bristol BS3 2NA
Telephone 0454 620070

MacWorld
IDG Communications
99 Gray's Inn Road
London WC1X 8UT
Telephone 071 831 9252

When you start using computers it is worth reading the associated technical journals. Don't be put off by the jargon — you will get used to it. These journals are full of tips and explanations but they are also a reminder of when an upgrade is due. If you act on the latter quickly enough you can save yourself money. Never rely on the vendors to keep you informed about upgrades.

Summary

Decide what you want a computer for. Get some background, read the journals. Ask around, especially get advice from those working in similar fields. Don't be fooled by vendors out for a quick sale. Purchase hardware which can be extended later. Separate units are better than a combined one. Go wild and spend enough to start with and you won't regret it. Make sure you get enough memory. Go for simplicity. ClarisWorks™, for example, will do all that many scientists need. Work through the tutorials that come with the program with courage, fortitude and patience, and you won't need to go on an expensive course.

WORKING METHODS   3

Controlling the factory — organising your filing system. What are the differences between folders, files and documents? Naming your documents. The Scrapbook and its uses. Saving and back-ing-up. Loss of data and how to prevent it. Finding lost work. Data storage in a multi-user environment. Security of 'sensitive' material.

A factory at your fingertips

You have at your fingertips not just a powerful workstation but an entire complex of factories devoted to storing and sorting any information you care to put in; then, at your command, these factories will produce work to a very high standard. If treated with respect, the workforce never goes on strike! If it does go on strike, you risk losing precious data. A few simple precautions will prevent this.

The computer organises itself around its system folder. Inside this folder there is a host of sub-controlling programs which find what you are going to work on, store and sort incoming data, set up the printer, and in general remember all you have told the computer to do. All the programs that you ever want to work with must be able to operate from only *one* system and finder. This is vital to success. Having more than one driving system on your hard disc is a certain recipe for disaster. This advice is specific to the Macintosh. Otherwise what follows is largely true for the MS-DOS environment also.

The system folder

On rare occasions, your computer may bomb out while doing a task. This is often the result of careless finger-work on your part, or of not reading or understanding the manual, i.e. you have asked it to do something it is not designed to do. Occasionally

Reasons for loss of data

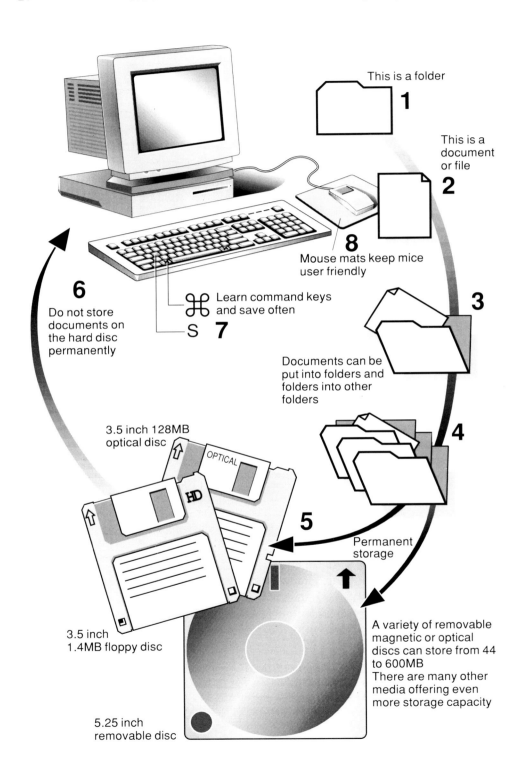

This is a folder **1**

This is a document or file **2**

8
Mouse mats keep mice user friendly

6
Do not store documents on the hard disc permanently

⌘ Learn command keys and save often
S **7**

3

Documents can be put into folders and folders into other folders

4

3.5 inch 128MB optical disc

OPTICAL

HD

5

Permanent storage

3.5 inch 1.4MB floppy disc

A variety of removable magnetic or optical discs can store from 44 to 600MB
There are many other media offering even more storage capacity

5.25 inch removable disc

there may be physical damage to discs. Excess dust or humidity, for instance, can cause malfunctions of a hard disc. Electricity failure or sudden surges can also lead to loss of data. Losing work after hours of labour is one of the most frustrating experiences known to computaholics and can lead to severe stress and suicidal tendencies!

Basic procedure

When you switch on your computer your screen will usually show icons for folders and documents and an icon representing the hard disc. This initial screen view is called the 'desktop'. To get organised we suggest you do the following: open a new folder and give it a name such as the date, or a person's name if you are doing something for somebody, or a name such as 'Current Work'. You have now created a place you can save your work, even if only temporarily. At least you will know where to find recent work, and you can always move it to a final location and rename it later if need be. This procedure can be performed before you start using a program. The next step is to open a program and start work but before you get going, if the work is new, perform the 'Save as...' task. This forces you to name the document or file you are working on so that it cannot get lost — anything with a name can always be found again. Some sort of housekeeping plan such as this, observed with discipline day after day, will save endless aggravation later. Get into the habit of using the command and 'S' keys often. This saves your work as you proceed.

Take no risks — save and back-up often

Disasters can be prevented if you perform the 'Save' procedure at *least* every ten minutes, but if you are doing work of a complex nature then save every five minutes or whenever a particular section has been completed. *Always* save the work before printing, and *always* save work before leaving the computer unattended, for however short a time.

In multi-user situations where, for instance, several people are feeding data into a single database, the saving routine must be very strictly observed. There are two good ways of ensuring this. One is to use programs that include an automatic save facility. This can be set to operate at a predetermined time. Or, designate one person to be responsible for supervision. This person then has to ensure that no machine is switched off until a check has been made and documents saved in the recommended manner.

Always back-up your data by making copies on floppy discs. This is best done on completion of each work session and certainly must be done at the end of the day. For long term storage of data, you may want to consider other storage media.

If disaster does strike, there are special rescue and first-aid programs which may enable you to recover work even after your computer has told you that all is lost. It is well worth investing in one of these.

Naming your documents

Naming documents properly is vital for all subsequent 'Save' operations, for all 'Find' operations (see below), and for your own convenience as well as that of others. We use the word 'properly' because experience has shown that some clever people like to use privately invented codes which they themselves subsequently forget and which are totally unintelligible to others when work is handed on. If you are working on 'Hormones', then at least designate the main storage folder with this title so that your colleagues can find it and use it. If you want to be secretive about it, then use FolderBolt™ (more below). The computer is intelligent enough to alert you if you try to use an identical name for more than one document or folder. Names have to be unique to each item saved.

Ways of identification Identification by date, as well as by name of person or project, can be a very helpful retrieval device. We suggest a simple numeric for dates: 051294, for example, would mean the 5th of December 1994. In some countries the day and month are reversed. This doesn't matter so long as work remains local. It can become important if you send data on disc to colleagues who use a different convention — you have to let them know which convention you are using. Slashes and full stops between numbers simply add complexity and may sometimes be misleading. The use of a hyphen as in the following example can be helpful: 120592-5. This could indicate that there are five documents belonging to the job. The important thing is to devise a method that suits you and to use it consistently.

Filing

You need to see that your factory is well-disciplined and orderly so that you can make the best use of your valuable time. If you follow the suggestions above, your documents will be properly filed in appropriate folders and will always be retrievable, just as in a conventional office. Should you forget where you've filed a document, there is a 'Find' instruction in the menu bar that tells the computer to make a search. This will always be successful, *provided* that you have given all your folders and documents unique names as mentioned above.

Folders on a computer behave exactly as folders do in reality: they are containers for documents. Individual jobs can be held in a named folder. Inside this folder there may be other folders. Unlike physical filing cabinets, computers can store folders inside folders ad infinitum, and this is very useful.

We stress that is advisable to set up a folder for a new job *before* starting the work. To do so is a distinct advantage because the computer is then able to file all subsequent work into the relevant folder at the touch of a button and you are less likely to lose the work and have to use 'Find'. If you have a folder entitled 'Current Work' on the desktop, i.e. visible in the window, then when you switch your computer on, it is particularly easy to access.

The Macintosh, Power PC and IBM are able to print out a catalogue of the current contents of each disc, and of each folder on that disc, as part of their standard procedures. This will enable you to keep a physical list of documents. If you choose to do this, it may be important to update it regularly. The hardcopy is also an insurance if the digital version is accidentally destroyed. *Catalogue of contents*

Documents and files are the same thing. The icon is a single page with the corner turned down (see the illustration on page 24), which denotes work done and saved. This may be just one page or hundreds. The work can be of any kind — drawings, texts, graphs, spreadsheets or databases — and could have been generated by any number of different programs.

Storage

If you are in a multi-user situation, then each department or unit within your working group should be assigned a storage disc for themselves. If the department is a large one with several subsections, then each of these may be allocated a disc. It could also be that if particular people are demanding a lot of work then they too will get their own disc. Don't be mean with storage discs. It is much safer to have many rather than try to cram everyone's work on to one disc. Experience has shown that one false manoeuvre can lose a lot of people's data.

For this reason, copying discs to form a backup set is also an important aspect of organisation. There are many storage devices on the market and you will need to find the method that is most suitable for your situation. An individual working at home, for instance, does not escape from the need to back-up data, but in this case it may be sufficient just to have enough double or high density floppies available for the purpose.

The computer hard disc should only be used for the storage of programs and as a temporary pool for the jobs you are currently working on. This means that your floppy discs become backup copies until you complete the jobs and return the work to these storage discs. To store immense amounts of valuable data on the computer hard disc is courting trouble. If this disc 'goes down', the work on it is often irrecoverable. But this isn't the only disadvantage. A hard disc used in this manner becomes increasingly fragmented and gets slower and slower. There are some programs that make temporary use of hard disc memory, so it is best to keep as much memory 'free' on the hard disc as you can.

There are three other storage facilities on all Macintosh and Power PC computers. The first is the 'Scrapbook'. This stays in the computer's memory even when the machine is switched off. Here you can store any frequently used items, be they drawings, texts or numeric data. Examples are: a quotation, a formula, family tree symbols, your letterhead logo. We mention the Scrapbook in many places throughout this book because it is so useful. (The Scrapbook facility does not currently exist on IBM machines.) The second storage possibility is to use the Library facility offered by some programs. The third possibility is to create a 'Stationery' pad for often-used items. Letterheads are an obvious example, but you can also keep any other document as a stationery pad, such as a basic drawing or chart which you will use and modify over and over again.

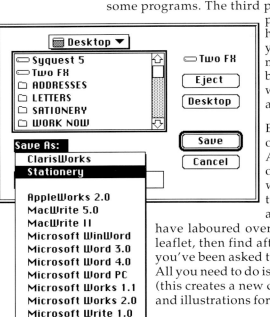

Efficient use of computers depends on not doing the same work twice. Any or all of the above storage methods can be used to help produce work quickly. Yet another method is to use previously created documents as templates for new ones. You may have laboured over the production of an information leaflet, then find after a while that it was so successful you've been asked to produce more in the same format. All you need to do is use the first one, rename and save it (this creates a new document), then exchange old texts and illustrations for new ones.

These are the 'save' options from ClarisWorks™ version 2. 'Stationery' is one of the choices. The 'desktop' window offers folders currently available for storage on the desktop

Security

There are several security programs on the market, such as FolderBolt™. This program allows you to customise the way you want your security system to operate. You can restrict the use of a computer to certain specified applications (programs), or to designated folders, or to stop intruders having access to the system folder and or finder folder. There is also a method of configuring what are called 'drop files' which allow the computer user to deposit data into a file without being able to open it. FolderBolt™ can be configured to work in almost any manner you like. Passwords may be used to allow access by certain people then changed once this permission has expired. If you assign a password to a document or folder make sure you don't forget it, otherwise you will never be able to access that data again! There are many security programs on the market but FolderBolt™ has a good reputation.

Summary

Create a special 'Current Work' folder for temporary storage on the desktop. Create a separate folder for each subject or person you deal with. Whenever you create a new document, save it as a named item, giving it a *unique* name. This is vital. Retrieval and search procedures depend on it. Save your work regularly and often. This means *at least* every ten minutes, and especially before printing or leaving the computer unattended. For any important documents, make sure that you create a backup copy immediately on a floppy disc. It's wise to do this twice for very vital material. Get to understand and use the various storage methods that are available. Keep the hard disc as 'clean' and uncluttered as possible. This will keep it running efficiently and save on memory.

PRINCIPLES OF LAYOUT AND TYPOGRAPHY

4

Good design makes for easy communication. Designing for a purpose and an audience. Legibility and readability. Page sizes, binding methods and margins. The anatomy of type and type-faces. Proportional and monospaced letterforms. Type styles, sizes and the mixing of type variants. Type and its background. Letter and word spacing. The measure or line length. Justified and flush-left settings. Line spacing or linefeed. Rules and under-lines. Grids: a way of organising a layout.

Why is design important?

The purpose of presenting any piece of information, whether it be displayed in the form of a handout, a report, a slide or a poster, is presumably that it will be read and remembered. The quality of the design affects reading and remembering in several ways.

Some of your audience may have the option of choosing whether or not to read what you are presenting. If the display is badly de-signed, the chances are they'll decide not to bother. If they are forced to bother because they need the information, it will take them longer than necessary to grasp the important points, there is a chance that they will misread or misunderstand them, and they are likely to remember less than they would with a well-designed display.

What is good design?

Good design is not just a matter of making marks in a way that you happen to find aesthetically pleasing. When you are design-ing information you are designing not for yourself but for your audience, and you are designing something that is intended to perform a specific function. The function of the display is the most important factor in determining what it should look like.

Good designers make sure that they fully understand the constraints imposed by function before they begin to design.

If you want your display to fulfil its function you must do the following:

- Consider convenience of use when choosing the physical form of the display.
- Make sure that the information content is appropriate for your audience.
- Ensure that the structure and sequence of the information is clearly shown.
- Present information in digestible amounts.
- Keep the display simple and uncluttered.
- Check that everything in the display is legible from the appropriate reading distance.

Now you can ask, 'Is it attractive?'. But just what is attractiveness? What makes things easy on the eye? A page that contains relevant information presented in a form that is both legible and easy to follow will be attractive for those very reasons. This may well be because of certain basic principles underlying the way in which we try to make sense out of what we see. Psychologists believe that we have a natural urge to look for groupings or patterns within an image. If there are unambiguous groupings or patterns, the brain is free to move on to the next problem; if there are no obvious patterns, we are often left with feelings of unease and dissatisfaction.

Good design uses type and space in such a way that there are unambiguous groupings of text elements on the page. Poor design creates ambiguous groupings so that the brain cannot reach a final conclusion about what is supposed to go with what. The result is uncomfortable and not aesthetically pleasing.

Over the centuries, certain principles for typography and layout have been established by typographers and printers. These basic principles are the subject of this chapter. They relate to aesthetic values and to legibility, and the value of many of them has been confirmed in this century by legibility research. They have thus been truly tried and tested, so you should never be tempted to ignore them just to be different.

Purpose, audience and mode of use

Under this heading we are mainly concerned with documents such as books and reports. Posters, slides and OHP transparencies are each dealt with in specific chapters later.

Remembering the importance of function, before you begin to design any kind of document you must consider the following questions:

* What kind of document is being proposed?
* Who is it for?
* How do you expect your readers or audience to use it?

You must also bear in mind the production method. Is the final printout to be from your wordprocessed text or will you use a page make-up program for a more professional touch? If the latter is the case then wordprocessing is only an intermediate step and does not itself require a sophisticated layout (see Chapter 12).

When you are planning a document, consider the motivation of your potential readers. The less well-motivated they are, the more important it is that the document should be attractive. Once it has been picked up and is in the hand of the reader, the author's case is almost won. If it remains on the table with all the other unattractive paper-junk, the relevance and clarity of the contents are immaterial. Here are some examples. **What kind of document is it?**

A novel usually inspires high reader motivation, perhaps because the cover is attractive, the title is intriguing, the author is well-known or one of your favourites, or you enjoy the genre. Novels are therefore not as dependent on attractive design as on content. The principal design features are legible type and a layout that is economic so that fewer pages are consumed and the book is therefore lighter and easier to hold. The binding should be such that the book opens easily and does not require two hands, yet does not fall to pieces at the slightest touch as so many paperbacks do. The optimum reading distance for hand-held material is about 30-40cm (12 to 15in). **A novel**

Instruction manuals have fair reader motivation. You do want to learn how your newly purchased widget works, even though you instinctively fix it together and press all the knobs before reading the instructions. Here the layout of the text is important. Instruction manuals need to be highly visual, with plenty of straightforward illustrations and precise, simple text broken into short, convenient sections. You need to be able to find reference to the relevant part of your widget easily and immediately without having to search a lengthy prose description. Manuals need to be bound so that they can open flat, bearing in mind that they may need to be used on a work bench while you are using both your hands to fix the wrongly assembled widget. The optimum reading distance may rise to as much as 60cm (24in), with a corresponding need to consider setting the text in a larger typeface. **An instruction manual**

Reference books inspire fair motivation because you have to learn in order to complete or achieve something else. Travel time- **A reference book** tables, log tables, standard meter settings, telephone directories: any of these may be needed to do your work. Here the layout becomes even more important, and complex reference works are often best designed by a specialist. This kind of material needs to be set economically to save printing costs, yet it must be easy to scan for the items you want. There are several design tricks that can be used to make horizontal scanning easier, for example, printing a pale background colour behind every other line of text.

A report Reports often have very low reader motivation because they are read as a duty rather than through choice. We are all tired of reports, and fully expect them to be boring. Unfortunately many scientific papers fall into this category. For any given subject, the specialist readers who will be fascinated and delighted with what you have written may be few. The vast majority will read your paper because it is their duty to keep up with what is going on. You could say that good design is more important for reports than for other kinds of printed materials. Readers may be attracted to a clear and inviting layout and find that, despite their fears, the content is interesting too.

Who is your Is your document for the elderly with a sight handicap; or chil-
document for? dren who have just learned to read; or students from another culture; or your peers who will be very familiar with your particular jargon; or the 'general' public — whoever they are? Communication and understanding are dependent not only on language but also on typography and layout.

How will your Will your document be referred to often; or be tucked away on a
document be shelf but used occasionally; or be read once and thrown away?
used? Even though the life of the document itself may be short, the information may be vital, thus justifying the time spent on the design. The manner and circumstances of use often affect the choice of binding method, and therefore the entire layout.

Legibility and readability

Eye movements To understand legibility, it helps to know a little about what hap-
in reading pens when we read. Rather than moving smoothly from left to right along each line, the eyes make a series of very rapid movements or 'saccades', pausing for about a quarter of a second between each movement to make a 'fixation'. Meaningful words such as nouns and verbs tend to be fixated more often than function words such as 'and'. About 94 per cent of reading time is spent on fixations, and the rest on saccades. If we encounter a problem, for example if a word is badly printed, or is unfamiliar to us, then we make a 'regression' — a backward saccade so that we can have another look. At the end of each line, the eyes make a 'backsweep' to the beginning of the next line. The accuracy of this

movement depends very much on the length of the lines of text and the amount of space between them.

At a normal reading distance, the image of perhaps three or four letters falls on the fovea, the part of the retina that has the highest visual acuity. In general, though, we are able to read three or four words at a time rather than three or four letters because we also make use of our peripheral vision. The number of letters or words that we are able to read at each fixation is known as the visual span, and it is affected by a number of typographic factors, as we shall see.

Exactly how we recognise letters and words is still not fully understood. Individual letters are probably identified by certain distinctive features that distinguish them from other letters. It is interesting that if a word in lowercase roman letters is cut in half horizontally, the word can be more easily recognised from the upper half than the lower half. This must be because the upper parts of the letters carry more distinctive features than the lower halves. *Recognising letters and words*

attributes of legibility

Research has shown that skilled readers recognise whole words at a time, but it is not certain whether they are treating the word as a single shape or recognising all of the individual letters simultaneously. But no matter how recognition comes about, bad typography will make it more difficult.

The word 'legibility' is used to mean the ease with which the text can be read. This has to do with the appearance of the text rather than its content. *Legibility*

Legibility is affected by such factors as:

- Type size.
- Typeface and type style.
- Spacing between letters and words.
- The length of the lines of text, called the 'measure'.
- The vertical distance between the lines of text, called line spacing or linefeed.
- The use and misuse of colour and tinted backgrounds.
- Paper quality and colour.
- Quality of copies.

- Ambient lighting. (The designer cannot control this but may have to take it into account, especially when designing posters.)

There are well-established design principles relating to these and other factors, as described in this chapter.

In its broadest sense, legibility also includes the ease with which the structure of the material can be grasped. This aspect of legibility depends on factors such as the appropriate use of spatial and typographic cueing, the use of rules (drawn lines), and the way text, tables and illustrations are placed in relation to one another. These issues are dealt with in Chapter 5.

Readability 'Readability' is usually used to refer to the ease with which the text can be understood. This depends on the way it is organised and worded. There are 'readability formulae', based on word length and sentence length, that can be used to assess reading ease, but there are many important aspects of writing that they do not take into account. The books listed under 'Further reading' on page 185 will help if you want to improve your writing.

If they are to function properly, your documents must be both legible and readable. The clearest text can be made incomprehensible by poor design. On the other hand, good design cannot compensate for badly organised or badly written text.

Page size

Before you can begin to design your document, you must know the page size. There are three series of paper sizes that are recommended jointly by the British Standards Institution and the International Organisation for Standardisation (BS 4000 : Part 1 : 1990; Part 2 : 1983). The 'A' series is intended for books, reports and stationery, and the 'B' series primarily for posters and magazines. The 'C' series relates to envelopes designed to take the A series of paper sizes. The A sizes are now widely used for publications of all kinds. A4 and A5 are the most popular for leaflets, booklets, reports and so on.

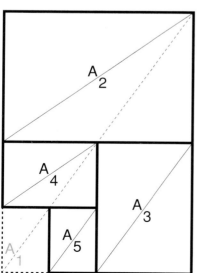

This is how the 'A' sizes of paper are related. A4 is used for many journals, reports and scientific documents. It is a size common to most of the 'desktop' printers. Some parts of the world such as USA (and other developing countries!) still use foolscap or 'legal' sizes. These sizes can cause difficulties when being photocopied or scanned because it is possible to lose data at the edges

If you are preparing a journal article or a book, your publisher may specify a non-A size, but if you have the choice we suggest that you use A sizes. Almost all printing companies are equipped to handle them, and they make for ease of storage and postage. There is scope for variation, for example by folding an A4 sheet into three, thus creating a leaflet with six columns of text when printed front and back. The A-size proportion (approximately 2:3) is also recommended for slides, OHP transparencies and microfiche, so use of these sizes allows easier transfer of information from one medium to another.

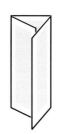

The design principles that we advise apply to the organisation of space whatever its shape, but for convenience we will consider the layout of text and illustrations on an A4 (210 x 297mm or 8.3 x 11.7in) sheet in the vertical format. Vertical formats are usually easier to file, shelve and bind than are horizontal formats.

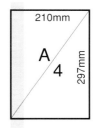

After page size, the next constraint is set by the binding method and this, in turn, usually determines the size of the margins.

Binding methods

In choosing a binding method, consider whether it would be helpful to be able to add, remove or replace pages. If so, you will want a form of loose-leaf binding rather than a permanent binding. You should also decide whether it is important that the publication should open flat, and what degree of strength is required in the binding. Cost is likely to be a factor too. The most common binding methods are summarised below.

Loose-leaf methods include the following:

Loose-leaf methods

- Single pages stapled in one corner simply to keep the pages together and in the right order.
- Single sheets in a ring binder. The document opens flat.
- Single pages in a plastic grip spine. The document will not open flat.
- Single pages in a plastic comb binding. The document opens flat.

These are commonly used permanent binding methods:

Permanent methods

- Double-page spreads stapled along a fold to make a booklet (saddle stitched). The document opens flat.
- Single pages in a wire spiral binding. The document opens flat.
- Single pages, with the back-edge glued into a spine within covers. This can be done professionally (called 'perfect binding'), or with a DIY machine (hot melt). The DIY method

looks professional but is not always easy to do well — pages can sometimes come unstuck. The document will not open flat.

- Single pages stapled from the side and glued into a cover (side stitched). This is a professional method, much used for glossy magazines. The document will not open flat.

- Double-page spreads, grouped into sections and sewn together, and then glued into a cover (section sewn). A professional method, this is the strongest and most permanent binding. The document will open more or less flat.

The choice of binding method will determine the minimum size of the back-edge margin. In general, methods that prevent the document from opening flat require a more generous back-edge margin. Remember, though, that if you are using a ring binder the margin must be wide enough for the punched holes to be well clear of the text area.

Margins

The minimum size of the back-edge margin is determined by the binding method, but the other margins cannot be finally decided on until you have made a number of other decisions.

Depending on the kind of information that you are dealing with, you may decide to treat the area of the page within the margins (the text area) as a single column or as two or more columns. This will affect the line length. The range of acceptable line lengths will in turn depend on your choice of typeface and type size. To achieve a suitable line length, you may have to adjust the margins, or even change the number of columns. Each choice affects the others and you may need to make several tests before you achieve a satisfactory result. All of these factors are discussed later in this chapter.

Back-edge margin If the back-edges of the sheets are fixed to a spine or firm binding there is always some limitation on the way the document opens. The back-edge margin must be wide enough to allow material at the edge of text area to be read easily without forcing the binding. We would strongly recommend that a model of the document be made, using the proposed binding method, to check on this problem before planning goes too far. Some universities, for example, specify a standard 38mm (1.5in) minimum margin on the lefthand edge for all thesis work. (Theses are typed only on one side of each sheet, so it's always the lefthand edge.)

Top and bottom margins The top and bottom margins are often the places where readers can be reminded which section of the document they are in, and where the author's name, the date and, most importantly, the

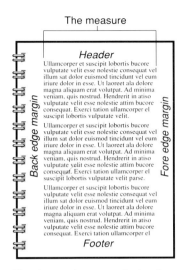

page number or other data that may have to run continuously from page to page are placed. This kind of information falls into a region outside the normal text area and is called a 'header' for the top margin and a 'footer' for the bottom margin. The bottom margin should be slightly greater than the top one, for several reasons. First, this is often where you need to hold the document. Second, it is aesthetically more pleasing to see the body of the text slightly raised on the page, especially if it is mostly continuous prose.

The fore-edge margin is often determined last, because it needs to be chosen so that the resulting line length is suitable for the type size. It may also be partially predetermined by the printing engine that is being used. Many laserprinters, for instance, require more margin space than other printing devices. ***Fore-edge margin***

With single-sided documents the back-edge margin will of course always be on the left and the fore-edge margin on the right. For double-sided printing it is important to remember that this situation will be reversed for lefthand pages.

Finally, do remember that a densely-packed page with the narrowest possible margins will look extremely uninviting. Generous margins give the page a much more open and accessible appearance.

The anatomy of type

Important features of letters are the descenders and ascenders of the lowercase letters, and the spaces, called 'counters', within certain letters and numerals. The strokes making up the letters have a 'stroke width'. This may vary within the character or it may be constant.

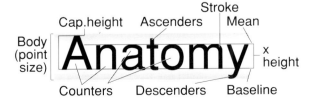

Type size is usually specified in points (a point is about one seventy-secondth of an inch). Unfortunately though, the type size in points is not a reliable guide to the height of the letters when printed. This is because the measurement relates to the 'body' of the type rather than to the letters themselves. In metal type, the body is the slug of metal on which the letter is cast. Electronic type has no physical body, but the same system of measurement has been adopted. As a result, examples of the same letter in the same point size but in different typefaces may differ considerably in size when printed. For this reason, type size can often be more usefully described in terms of capital letter height and x-height.

Typefaces

There are two major groups of typefaces, those with serifs and those without. Serifs are the finishing shapes at the ends of the strokes, and it is said that they aid legibility by helping to guide the eyes along each line. This may be true, because if we can visually group parts of an image to form a smooth, continuous line, then we will do so. Psychologists call this 'good continuation'. The serifs at the base of a line of letters may therefore create a horizontal emphasis which helps to guide the eye. Serifs may also contribute to the recognition of individual letters. The majority of books are printed using serifed typefaces, so they certainly have the advantage of familiarity.

Sans serif style

T 3

Monoline stroke

Serif style

T 3

Variable stroke

Most, but not all, serifed faces have a variable stroke width. The variation may be slight or it may be marked. Most, but not all, sans serif faces have a constant stroke width and are described as 'monoline' faces.

Anatomy
Anatomy

So which typefaces are best? This depends to a large extent on the function of the document. Long passages of unbroken prose may be easier to read when a serifed typeface is used, but texts that are liable to be photocopied and re-photocopied (see left) through several generations are best not set in a serifed typeface. The thin strokes may soon disappear, making nonsense of the words. Serifed faces often create difficulties for photographers too, especially when blue diazo slides are required. Sans serif styles have a bolder, businesslike feel about them, but are best kept for shorter chunks of text. Sans serif typefaces are ideal for illustrations, particularly if they might also be used for slides.

Proportional versus monospaced letterforms

Monospaced letterforms were designed for early models of manual typewriters. The characters all have the same 'body' width, so an 'm' will look cramped and an 'i' will appear to be surrounded by too much space. Monospaced letterforms are still used for some impact printers, mainly of the daisywheel variety.

Your computer system should offer at least one monospaced typeface in addition to its proportionally-spaced faces. There may be several good reasons for using a monospaced typeface; for example:

- To enable you to match new texts with older monospaced versions.

- To make certain kinds of work easier by allowing consistent vertical alignment, such as in amino acid sequences.

- In some circumstances it is easier to calculate the length of a document.

The three fonts shown here are in the *same* point size

Times Roman has proportional spacing, which makes it impossible to align the hyphens under one another

Arg-Phe-Asp-
His-Gln-Met-

Courier is the only monospaced typeface supplied with your printer. Its rather thin strokes don't work well on slides and it takes up more horizontal space than Times

Arg-Phe-Asp-
His-Gln-Met-

Helmono is a monospaced font based on Helvetica™ which works successfully for slides. (See page 188 for details of how to obtain this font)

Arg-Phe-Asp-
His-Gln-Met-

It is as well to remember that all monospaced letterforms are inherently harder to read because of their relatively crude spacing, and more difficult to photograph or photocopy because they are rather 'thin'. Remember too that a monospaced face always occupies more paper area than a similar proportionally-spaced face.

Type styles

Each typeface is normally available in a number of styles. In science we are primarily concerned with the use of bold and italic since these two styles are used so much for citing references and for foreign words. Once again, bold or italic lettering must be used with care when designing work for diazo slides because

Bold and italic

they may seriously impair legibility. The counters in either of these styles may fill in and cause words to become illegible in some circumstances.

Normal
Italic
Bold

Bold is best avoided for continuous text because its heavy texture can produce afterimages that cause the white spaces between and within the letters to glow and vibrate. It is extremely useful for emphasis though, as we shall see in Chapter 5. Italics reduce reading speed when used for continuous text, but there is no reason why they shouldn't be used to distinguish small amounts of text.

Condensed type Condensed styles can be very useful where space is limited, as in telephone directories for example, but it is essential that the reproduction should be of a high standard. If it is not, there is a risk that the counters will fill in and that adjacent letters will run together. With materials that are read at a distance, such as slides and posters, the white spaces within and between letters may appear to fill in, even if the images are of a high quality. It is therefore safer to avoid condensed styles unless you have a compelling reason for using them.

Condensed
Extended

Extended type Extended styles tend to reduce legibility simply because they occupy more horizontal space than type of normal proportions. This means that the reader is able to perceive fewer letters and words at each fixation of the eyes, so more fixations are required and reading time is increased. The additional space occupied is in itself a disadvantage in many situations, but extended type can be useful in small quantities for display purposes.

Outline and Shadow Outline and Shadow styles are best avoided. In small sizes they are fatal for legibility, especially where photocopying or photography are involved. They also tell the world that your document has been desktop-published rather than professionally typeset.

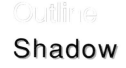

Shadow

Underlines The 'underline' feature of many wordprocessing programs is derived from the design of traditional typewriter letterforms and is always far too close to the descenders. Underlining is merely an effective way of reducing legibility by consuming essential inter-line space. Never use this feature. It is more elegant to avoid underlining altogether and instead use the other typographic facilities at your disposal, such as italic or bold.

Typestyle
Typestyle

(Note: If you wish to separate text from other material below it, then the correct way to do this is by drawing in a 'rule'; see the last example on the previous page.)

Text set in all-capital letters takes longer to read than text set in a mixture of capitals and lowercase letters. This is mainly because the ascenders and descenders of the lowercase letters create much more distinctive and easily recognisable letter and word shapes than those produced by capital letters. Capital letters have the added disadvantage of taking up more space horizontally than lowercase letters of the same type size (see example (a) below). As a result, fewer words can be read at each fixation, so reading time is increased. The use of all-capital lettering is therefore best avoided, except possibly for short headings.

Capital letters versus lowercase letters

In scientific writing it is often necessary to use capitals for acronyms, abbreviations and symbols. In example (a) below, they are difficult to recognise. In example (b) they stand out clearly from other data, but they have more emphasis than they deserve. They destroy the even texture or 'colour' of the text. An elegant solution to this problem is to use a smaller size of capital letters. A difference of two points will usually be sufficient to prevent acronyms and abbreviations from becoming an unnecessary distraction in the text. You will find that some typefaces have a special 'small caps' font: see example (c).

Small capitals

All of the examples below have been set in Helvetica™

a.   ALL TEXTS FOR CONTINUOUS READING SHOULD BE IN LOWERCASE CHARACTERS. CAPITALS SHOULD BE RESERVED FOR RECOGNISED ABBREVIATIONS SUCH AS THOSE USED IN CHEMISTRY: CO2. THE SAME APPLIES TO THE ACRONYMS OF WHICH EVERY SPECIALTY IS SO FOND, SUCH AS DSS, THE NHS, ACTH AND DNA, AND SO ON. NEVER MAKE THESE UP YOURSELF WITHOUT EXPLAINING THEM. PLACE NO ADDITIONAL STUMBLING BLOCKS IN THE PATH OF THE READER.

b.   All texts for continuous reading should be in lowercase characters. Capitals should be reserved for recognised abbreviations such as those used in chemistry: CO_2. The same applies to the acronyms of which every specialty is so fond, such as DSS, the NHS, ACTH and DNA, and so on. Never make these up yourself without explaining them. Place no additional stumbling blocks in the path of the reader.

c.   All texts for continuous reading should be in lowercase characters. Capitals should be reserved for recognised abbreviations such as those used in chemistry: CO_2. The same applies to the acronyms of which every specialty is so fond, such as DSS, the NHS, ACTH and DNA, and so on. Never make these up yourself without explaining them. Place no additional stumbling blocks in the path of the reader.

Type and its background

Reversed type For continuous reading, black type on a white background is more legible than white type on a black background. This is because small bright images on a dark background will appear to spread. For good legibility of reversed type it is important to use a typeface that has open counters, and to ensure that the letter spacing is not too tight. Sans serif faces are often more legible than serifed faces because serifed letters may appear to be joined by their serifs, especially in poor lighting. The legibility of white type on a black background will also suffer if the quality of reproduction is not good. Thin strokes may disappear, so a monoline sans serif face is likely to be more legible than a serifed face.

White-on-black type can be useful for headings and for drawing attention to short sections of text, provided that the above points are borne in mind.

White on black
White on black

Patterned Patterned backgrounds can severely reduce the legibility of any
backgrounds type placed over them. The pattern not only reduces the contrast between the type and its background; it can also affect the outlines of the letters and make them more difficult to recognise. The coarser the pattern, the greater the interference will be. Sans serif faces tend to be more legible than serifed faces because there are no fine serifs or delicate hairline strokes to be obliterated. Remember too that any background to a text may make it impossible to photocopy satisfactorily.

Black on tints
Black on tints

Sizes of type

The choice of type size must depend on the function of the text. It should never depend solely on the economics of trying to fit too much information into a limited space.

Your text will almost certainly fall into one of these groups:

- Notices to be read at a given distance.
- Poster presentations to be read at a given distance.
- Slides to be viewed at a given distance.
- Documents to be read on the bench top at a distance of 45-60cm (18-24in).
- Documents to be read at a distance of 30-40cm (12-15in).

Letter sizes for There is an easy way to calculate the optimum type size for post-
signs and ers or sign boards. The formula given here has been found to pro-
posters vide a working guide for the optimum lettering size for good legibility under 'normal' lighting conditions.

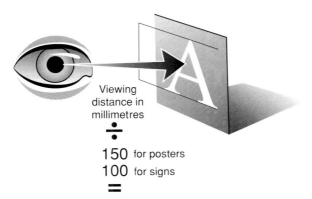

Viewing
distance in
millimetres

÷

150 for posters
100 for signs

=

actual minimum size of lettering in situ at
the reading distance specified by poster
organisers or the distance of the sign

For slides and OHPs, the table below gives the type size to use when the size of your artwork is fixed, and the artwork size for five different type sizes. Artwork based on this table will always produce legible results, provided there is sufficient contrast between the lettering and background.

Letter sizes for slides and OHPs

For paper sizes up to A4

Legible lettering calculator for OHP and slides

1 If you are limited to a particular type size, artwork should be kept within a rectangle of the size shown

2 If you draw within a given rectangle, use the type size shown

Rectangle of artwork area	Cap. height (Helvetica)
16 x 24cm (6.5 x 9.5in)	6mm or 24pt
13 x 20cm (8 x 5.25in)	5mm or 18pt
10.5 x 16cm (6.25 x 4.25in)	4mm or 14pt
8 x 12cm (3.25 x 4.75in)	3mm or 12pt
5 x 8cm (2.25 x 3.25in)	2mm or 10pt

The specification for type size given by most scientific journals is for a capital letter height of not less than 2mm for the final printed letter size. The capital letter height is used because point size is not an accurate predictor of final printed size. In the example on the right, all four characters are the *same* point size. Times Roman™ 12pt will give a capital letter height of about 2mm, but so will 10pt Palatino™. (See Glossary for an explanation of point sizes.)

Letter sizes for print

Courier　　Palatino

BBBB

Times　　Helvetica

In most printed documents the text size will be somewhere between 10pt and 12pt. Fourteen-point is a little large for normal documents, but 14pt to 18pt can be very useful for notes that may have to be referred to in a darkened lecture hall. Type sizes of 18pt and above are considered to be 'display' sizes.

Mixing typefaces and sizes

Documents that consist of a large variety of typefaces and sizes are characteristic of the amateur designer. You have an enormous choice of faces and sizes of type and it is essential that you use them just as you would use any other tool — choose the one that is appropriate for the job. There are people who will fix a cupboard on the wall by banging the screws in with a hammer rather than screwing them in with a screwdriver. The results of  using the wrong tool are usually dangerous; in typography they are merely confusing and ugly, but this will be sufficient to lose the interest of your audience.

By the time you have read this book and absorbed the information in it we hope you will be able to make informed decisions about typefaces. Times Roman™ is one of the most economic as well as one of the most legible of all typefaces. Bookman™, on the other hand, is generous and occupies plenty of space, and because the counters are full and open it is useful for 35mm slides. Helvetica™ has a relatively large x-height in relation to its capital letter height and it is therefore highly legible, particularly in difficult circumstances where lighting may be poor. Palatino™ is an 'elegant' typeface with rather longer descenders and ascenders; it is thus less economic than Times because it requires more space between lines, but its elegance makes it suitable for poetry or novels. Avant Garde™ is a 'difficult' typeface to use for texts because it is rather too generous in width. This is likely to reduce the visual span, thus increasing the number of fixations and hence the total reading time. However, the display sizes of Avant Garde™ can be useful because they are not as heavy as those of some other faces.

It is sometimes valuable to introduce a different typeface for headings, subheadings, quotes, or wherever you feel that a style variation has a definite message to convey. In this book we have used Palatino™ for all general text, including all headings and subheadings, and Helvetica™ for shoulder heads, chapter synopses, summaries, captions and illustration labels. If you want to mix typefaces in this way, make sure you use two faces that are

clearly different. Times Roman™ and New Century School-
book™, for example, are not dissimilar when used in normal text
sizes. The difference must be great enough not to appear acciden-
tal, or the reader won't be sure whether it has any significance or
not. The same principle applies to the use of more than one size.

Our message here is this: choose one typeface for your main text,
be it a hand-held document, 35mm slide, poster, OHP presentation or whatever. For headings within the text, use the same face
two sizes larger, or one size larger set in bold. Avoid all the fancy
variants like Outline and Shadow until you are more familiar
with the general principles of typography and graphic design.
The good designer knows how to keep it simple and employs the
discipline of a restricted choice. The bad designer doesn't know
when enough is enough.

Letter and word spacing

Letter and word spacing are normally dealt with automatically
by most wordprocessing programs, but there are times when control over the space between let-
ters and words becomes useful
and can improve legibility. This
is particularly true for words set
in display sizes. Bad automatic
spacing becomes especially apparent when capital letters are
used. Example (a) illustrates
equal spacing. There is too much
space between W and A, and A
and T. Example (b) is the same as
(a) with the lines removed. In (c) these letter pairs have been
'kerned' to reduce the space between them. Most wordprocessing
programs kern automatically where necessary. In page make-up
programs you will also have manual control of kerning.

(a) **WATER**

(b) **WATER**

(c) **WATER**

The space between words should approximate to the space that
would be occupied by an 'e' in the same font, placed as if it were
touching the letters before and after it. You have little control over
this in wordprocessing programs and total control over it in page
make-up programs. Unless you are going in for professional
typesetting, you will not need to be concerned with these issues.

If you are setting a piece of wordprocessed text that you did not
type, check to make sure that there is only one word space after
punctuation marks. Extra word spaces are likely to reduce legibility (see page 146), and they announce that your work has not
been professionally typeset. Extra spaces can also cause havoc
with optical character recognition (OCR) software.

***Spaces after full
stops***

Line length: the 'measure'

Short lines containing very few words prevent us from making efficient use of our peripheral vision when reading, so the normal pattern of eye movements is disrupted. Long lines, on the other hand, make it very difficult for the eyes to make an accurate back-sweep from the end of one line to the beginning of the next. Several fixations may be required before the correct place is found. It is therefore counterproductive to try to fit as much information as possible onto each page by using the maximum possible line length. Better use can be made of the page area by setting the text in two or more columns. This not only gives a more legible line length but also enables you to fit more text into the same print area.

The optimum length of line for continuous printed text has been variously described as minimum of 6 to a maximum of 10 words per line. But this is a rather inaccurate measure as many scientific and technical texts have a preponderance of long words. It is more accurate to count the number of characters per line. Each letter, numeral, punctuation mark or space is a 'character'. Research has shown that the optimum number of characters per line is about 60 to 70; 65 is a good number to aim for, and 70 should be taken as the upper limit. At the lower end of the range, lines of 40 to 50 characters are acceptable. The character count becomes very important when estimating the length of documents and the number of pages that the text will occupy.

Line length calculation Another useful rule-of-thumb is based on the length of the lower-case alphabet in the typeface and size you are using. The line length should be between 1.5 and 2.5 times the alphabet length, giving a character count of between 40 and 65. The longer the lines, the more important it is that there should be sufficient space between them. This helps readers to stay on the correct line and to find their way easily to the beginning of each new line.

For slides, posters, and other displays designed to be read from a distance, the line length should be not more than 1.5 times the alphabet length. This is because the lettering in these kinds of display is designed to be legible from the maximum likely viewing distance. When viewed from closer quarters, lines of even moderate length can seem very long. It can become a conscious effort to drag the eyes from the end of one line to the beginning of the next.

Since the optimum length of line for good legibility is defined in terms of numbers of characters, it follows that the optimum length in picas (see Glossary), inches or millimetres will depend on the typeface and type size chosen. With monospaced letterforms it is of course very easy to relate numbers of characters to line lengths in inches. With proportionally-spaced type you will need to do some sample settings in your chosen face and size to make sure that your proposed line length is acceptable.

Justified versus flush-left setting

With flush-left setting, also called ranged-left or unjustified setting, each line is filled to the nearest whole word. Letter and word spacing remain constant, so the righthand margin is uneven or 'ragged'. Hyphenation hardly exists, and when it does occur, it is usually restricted to very long words. With justified setting, all lines have the same length and both margins are even. This is achieved by varying the word spacing, and sometimes the letter spacing too. Most justification methods used by computers also include automatic hyphenation. The shorter the line, the more hyphenation there is.

The four margin settings available in most wordprocessing and page make-up programs. Note that a justified setting occupies fewer lines

1

1 Justified. Some wordprocessing programs lack sophisticated hyphenation procedures. Good hyphenation control is necessary if white islands and rivers are to be avoided

Lorem ipsum dolor sit amet, consectetuer adipiscing elit, sed diam nonummy nibh euismod tincidunt ut laoreet dolore magnam aliquam erat volutpat. Ut wisi enim ad minim veniam, quis nostrud exerci tation ullamcorper suscipit lobortis nislto ut aliquip ex ea commodo consequat. Duis autem veleum iriure dolorino hendrerit in vulputate velit essem molestie consequat, vel illum dolore eula feugiat nulla facilisis at vero eroset accumsan et iusto odio dignissim qui blandit praesent luptatum zril delenit augue duis dolore te feugait nulla facilisi.

2

Lorem ipsum dolor sit amet, consectetuer adipiscing elit, sed diam nonummy nibh euismod tincidunt ut laoreet dolore magnam aliquam erat volutpat. Ut wisi enim ad minim veniam, quis nostrud exerci tation ullamcorper suscipit lobortis nislto ut aliquip ex ea commodo consequat. Duis autem veleum iriure dolorino hendrerit in vulputate velit essem molestie consequat, vel illum dolore eula feugiat nulla facilisis at vero eroset accumsan et iusto odio dignissim qui blandit praesent luptatum zril delenit augue duis dolore te feugait nulla facilisi.

2 Flush-left. This can create a very ragged appearance, particularly if there are a lot of long words and the measure is short

3 Flush-right. This has the same raggedness problem and is also harder to read. It does sometimes have a use for short captions placed to the left of illustrations

3

Lorem ipsum dolor sit amet, consectetuer adipiscing elit, sed diam nonummy nibh euismod tincidunt ut laoreet dolore magnam aliquam erat volutpat. Ut wisi enim ad minim veniam, quis nostrud exerci tation ullamcorper suscipit lobortis nislto ut aliquip ex ea commodo consequat. Duis autem veleum iriure dolorino hendrerit in vulputate velit essem molestie consequat, vel illum dolore eula feugiat nulla facilisis at vero eroset accumsan et iusto odio dignissim qui blandit praesent luptatum zril delenit augue duis dolore te feugait nulla facilisi.

4

Lorem ipsum dolor sit amet, consectetuer adipiscing elit, sed diam nonummy nibh euismod tincidunt ut laoreet dolore magnam aliquam erat volutpat. Ut wisi enim ad minim veniam, quis nostrud exerci tation ullamcorper suscipit lobortis nislto ut aliquip ex ea commodo consequat. Duis autem veleum iriure dolorino hendrerit in vulputate velit essem molestie consequat, vel illum dolore eula feugiat nulla facilisis at vero eroset accumsan et iusto odio dignissim qui blandit praesent luptatum zril delenit augue duis dolore te feugait nulla facilisi.

4 Centred. This can be useful when limited to title pages and short texts, but text set in this manner is also not so easy to read

There is no such thing as 'justified right' or 'justified left'. These phrases are the result of ignorance, but unfortunately they do appear in some manuals.

For many people, justification has a certain amount of prestige value because it is the way in which most books, magazines and newspapers are set. However, we know of no research that has shown justified setting to be more legible than flush-left setting. Most researchers have been unable to find any difference between them, and indeed some studies have suggested a slight advantage in favour of unjustified setting for less skilled readers and very short lines.

The problem with justified setting is that the irregular letter and word spacing becomes very noticeable with shorter line lengths. The text becomes uneven in appearance, with word spaces creating a powerful pattern of vertical white rivers which the reader will be unable to ignore. Rivers and ugly spaces are especially common in the ultra-narrow columns of daily newspapers. This occurs very easily when the number of words per line drops below six. There may also be an unacceptably large number of hyphenations.

Lorem ipsum dolor sit amet, consectet er adipiscing elit, sed diam nonummy nibh-euismod tincidunt ut laoreet dolore magna aliquam erat volutpat. Ut wisi enim ad-mini veniam, quis nostrud exerci tation ullamcorper-suscipit lobo ertis nisl ut aliquip exea commodo consequat. Duis autem vel-eum iriure dolor in hendrerit in vulputate velit esse molestie consequat, vel illum dolore eu feugiat nulla facilisis at vero eros et accumsan et iusto odio-dignissim qui blandit praesent lupta tum zril delenit augue du dolore te-feugait nulla

Many wordprocessing programs cannot cope with very short lines. In the example here, the number of words per line drops below the threshold of six and ugly white rivers can be seen. You will have to experiment with your own program to find out how many words per line are needed for an acceptable result

Since there is likely to be no real difference in the legibility of justified and flush-left setting when typeset in line lengths of more than 50 or so characters and spaces, the decision can then rest on other factors. From an aesthetic point of view it can be argued that flush-left setting avoids the slab-like appearance of justified text, but there may be occasions when a straight righthand margin seems more appropriate. On a more practical note, flush-left setting causes the text to occupy more space than justified setting.

It is generally agreed that flush-right and centred setting severely reduce legibility. The lines begin at different points, so it will be more difficult for the eyes to find the beginning of each new line. These settings are therefore not suitable for continuous text, but they may sometimes be appropriate for small quantities of text or for displayed headings.

Line spacing (linefeed)

When you have selected a point size for your type, your word-processing or page make-up program will need to know how much space you require between lines. Your program may refer to 'line spacing', 'linefeed' or 'inter-line spacing'. In some software the word 'leading' is used to mean linefeed, but this is not the correct use of the term (see Glossary).

Helvetica 10pt on 10pt linefeed (set solid)

Helvetica 10pt on 12pt linefeed

Lorem ipsum dolor sit amet, consectetuer adipiscing elit, sed diam nonummy nibhil to euismod tincidunt ut laoreet dolore magna aliquam erat volutpat. Ut wisi enim add minim veniam, quis nostrud exercitation ullam corper via suscipit lobortis nisl ut nuter aliquip ex ea commodo bol consequat. Duis autem vel eum iriure dolor in hendrerit.

Lorem ipsum dolor sit amet, consectetuer adipiscing elit, sed diam nonummy nibhil to euismod tincidunt ut laoreet dolore magna aliquam erat volutpat. Ut wisi enim add minim veniam, quis nostrud exercitation ullam corper via suscipit lobortis nisl ut nuter aliquip ex ea commodo bol consequat. Duis autem vel eum iriure dolor in hendrerit.

Note that because of the short lines we have had to set these texts flush-left in order to avoid rivers

Linefeed is measured from baseline to baseline. If you have chosen, say, 10pt type, a 10pt linefeed will be sufficient to prevent ascenders and descenders on adjacent lines from touching, but most typefaces benefit from a little more space between lines. You might, therefore, choose an 11pt linefeed for your 10pt type. If your program has an 'auto-leading' option, this will probably give you a linefeed of 120% of the type size, so if you are using 10pt type you will have a 12pt linefeed. It is much better, though, to choose a linefeed that is appropriate for the typeface and line length that you are using, as we explain below.

When you are trying to calculate how many lines of type will fit onto a page, it is the linefeed that you need to know rather than the point size of the type. If you want to find out what the linefeed is on an existing piece of text, the most accurate and convenient way of measuring it is with a typescale.

How much space? So how much inter-line space is needed? The white space between lines should always be greater than the space between words. This will ensure that words are visually grouped into lines, thus helping the eyes to follow each line rather than slipping down to the next. Adequate line spacing also makes it easier to find the beginning of each new line.

As a rule-of-thumb, the minimum spacing between lines of normal prose, measured from the baseline of one line of lettering to the baseline of the next, should be about 1.5 times the capital letter height. This is not the ideal way of deciding on line spacing however. Some typefaces have longer ascenders and descenders than others, so measuring the capital letter height alone can lead to errors.

As suggested above, one or two additional points of space will always improve legibility. This is especially true for:

• Line lengths approaching the upper limit for good legibility.

• Faces with a relatively large x-height in relation to the capital letter height.

The amount of space must be proportional to the size of the type. For example, if 10pt type needs 2 points of additional space, then 14pt will need 3 points. Too much space will reduce legibility, however.

Subscripts and superscripts Subscripts and superscripts can cause special problems with line spacing. It is important that they shouldn't touch the type on the line above or the line below, so you may need to increase the linefeed to prevent this. For consistency you must increase the linefeed throughout your document, so ideally you should be able to adjust it in 1pt increments so that it does not become unnecessarily large. If you don't add enough extra space, you may find that your wordprocessing program automatically increases the linefeed for those lines containing subscripts or superscripts. The resulting uneven line spacing is ugly and distracting.

H_2O

$125I$

H_2O

$125I$

Exceptions

There may be occasions when you just want to get words down on paper quickly without bothering with all this 'design palaver.' This might be true for last-minute lecture handouts or notes for a meeting. However, it is unwise to ignore the importance of using a suitable line length and sufficient space between lines. As the length of the text line increases, so the space between lines should increase proportionally. Even hastily prepared documents need a minimum standard of legibility.

Rules

Ruled lines in the right place can effectively divide or group parts of the text or illustrations. Rules should be thought of as a design feature in their own right and not as an adjunct to lettering.

Some wordprocessing programs do not have a horizontal line feature. The ability to draw lines either vertically or horizontally and of any thickness, toning or style, belongs mainly to page make-up, drawing or painting programs. For some purposes (in tables, for example) it is an advantage to be able to use rules of less than one point in thickness, so this may be a feature worth checking when you are choosing a wordprocessing program.

Use rules sparingly and favour horizontal stress rather than vertical. The reason for this is that the standard reading mode of 'western' cultures requires horizontal eye movements more often than vertical movements.

The grid — designing pages with their contents in columns

For a professional finish, the text must be consistently placed on each page. The same principle applies to the design of slides and poster displays. A reader who takes the time to look carefully should be able to see why each element is placed as it is. There should be no inexplicable random indents, or pieces of information that seem not to line up with anything else on the page. This consistency is achieved by the use of a grid. The grid defines the position of the margins, the text area, and any subdivisions of the text area.

In planning your grid, you have a choice between setting your text in one column, or in more than one column. This decision depends largely on the kind of information that is to be presented, but the number of columns must also be chosen in relation to the page size and the proposed type size. Dividing the text into more than one column may make it more legible. For example, you may decide to use a small type size for economic reasons and to make the document less bulky. But as the type gets smaller so the character count in the measure increases and at around 70 it becomes uncomfortable to read. A two-column layout is the answer. This is why many scientific journals are printed in this manner. Newspapers are designed with many columns because this provides editors with the greatest flexibility for manoeuvring stories about. Illustrations are easier to fit in too.

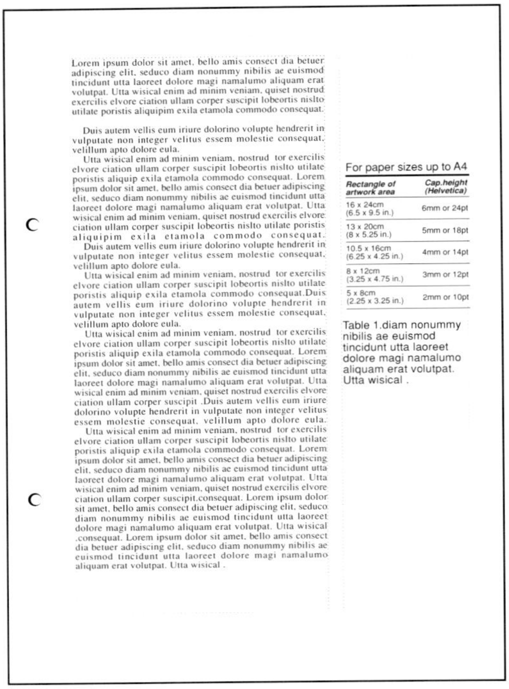

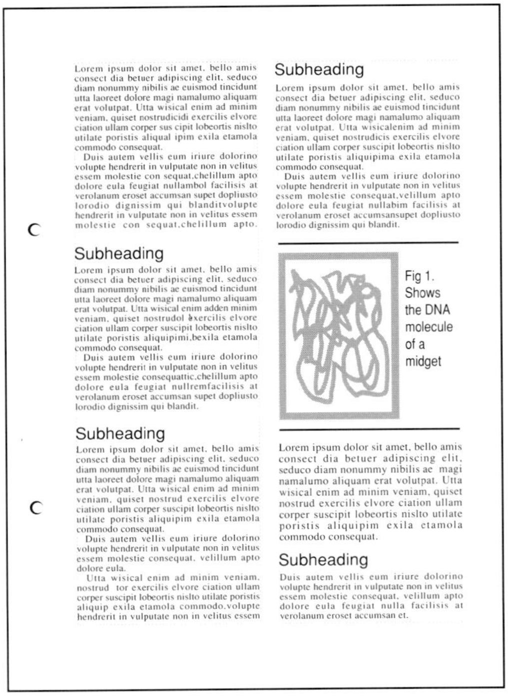

In many wordprocessing programs each column is the same pre-set width. Page make-up programs on the other hand may allow you to vary the column width to suit a specific purpose. An instruction manual, for instance, may work best if it has a narrow column for marginal shoulder notes, set in a small type size, with a much wider column for the general prose which will be set in a larger size.

Among the most frequently used grid structures are:

- A single column.
- Two asymmetric columns.
- Two symmetric columns.
- Three asymmetric columns.
- Three symmetric columns.

Single-column grids are suitable for documents that have few tables or illustrations, or where the tables and illustrations are all of the same width. They are economical in terms of the amount of text that can be fitted in, but they can be dull to look at. On an A4 page they can result in over-long lines , unless wide margins are used.

Two-column grids give more flexibility for publications containing tables and illustrations of different sizes. Asymmetric two-column grids (top left, this page) have a wider column and a narrower column, with the widths usually in some simple ratio such as 2:1 or 3:1. This gives a choice of three widths for tables and illustrations: they may occupy the wider column, the narrower column, or both. The narrower column can also be used for headings, captions or notes, as well as small illustrations. It is important, though, not to have too many different

---

Left column example box 1:

Lorem ipsum dolor sit amet, bello amis consect dia betuer adipiscing elit, seduco diam nonummy nibilis ae euismod tincidunt utta laoreet dolore magi namalumo aliquam erat volutpat. Utta wisical enim ad minim veniam, quiset nostrud exercilis elvore ciation ullam corper suscipit lobeortis nislto utilate poristis aliquipin exila etamola commodo consequat.

Duis autem vellis eum iriure dolorino volupte hendrerit in vulputate non integer velitus essem molestie consequat. velillum apto dolore eula.

Utta wisical enim ad minim veniam, nostrud tor exercilis elvore ciation ullam corper suscipit lobeortis nislto utilate poristis aliquip exila etamola commodo consequat. Lorem ipsum dolor sit amet, bello amis consect dia betuer adipiscing elit, seduco diam nonummy nibilis ae euismod tincidunt utta laoreet dolore magi namalumo aliquam erat volutpat. Utta wisical enim ad minim veniam, quiset nostrud exercilis elvore ciation ullam corper suscipit lobeortis nislto utilate poristis aliquipim exila etamola commodo consequat.

Duis autem iriure dolore non iriure hendrerit in vulputate non integer velitus essem molestie consequat. velillum apto dolore eula.

Utta wisical enim ad minim veniam, nostrud tor exercilis elvore ciation ullam corper suscipit lobeortis nislto utilate poristis aliquip exila etamola commodo consequat.Duis autem vellis eum iriure dolorino volupte hendrerit in vulputate non integer velitus essem molestie consequat. velillum apto dolore eula.

Utta wisical enim ad minim veniam, nostrud tor exercilis elvore ciation ullam corper suscipit .Duis autem vellis eum iriure dolorino volupte hendrerit in vulputate non integer velitus essem molestie consequat. velillum apto dolore eula.

Utta wisical enim ad minim veniam, nostrud tor exercilis elvore ciation ullam corper suscipit lobeortis nislto utilate poristis aliquip exila etamola commodo consequat. Lorem ipsum dolor sit amet, bello amis consect dia betuer adipiscing elit, seduco diam nonummy nibilis ae euismod tincidunt utta laoreet dolore magi namalumo aliquam erat volutpat. Utta wisical enim ad minim veniam, quiset nostrud exercilis elvore ciation ullam corper suscipit.consequat. Lorem ipsum dolor sit amet, bello amis consect dia betuer adipiscing elit, seduco diam nonummy nibilis ae euismod tincidunt utta laoreet dolore magi namalumo aliquam erat volutpat. Lorem ipsum dolor dia betuer adipiscing elit, seduco diam nonummy nibilis ae euismod tincidunt utta laoreet dolore magi namalumo aliquam erat volutpat. Utta wisical .

Inset table within box 1:

For paper sizes up to A4

Rectangle of artwork area	Cap.height (Helvetica)
16 x 24cm (6.5 x 9.5 in.)	6mm or 24pt
13 x 20cm (8 x 5.25 in.)	5mm or 18pt
10.5 x 16cm (6.25 x 4.25 in.)	4mm or 14pt
8 x 12cm (3.25 x 4.75 in.)	3mm or 12pt
5 x 8cm (2.25 x 3.25 in.)	2mm or 10pt

Table 1.diam nonummy nibilis ae euismod tincidunt utta laoreet dolore magi namalumo aliquam erat volutpat. Utta wisical .

Left column example box 2:

Lorem ipsum dolor sit amet, bello amis consect dia betuer adipiscing elit, seduco diam nonummy nibilis ae euismod tincidunt utta laoreet dolore magi namalumo aliquam erat volutpat. Utta wisical enim ad minim veniam, quiset nostrudicis exercilis elvore ciation ullam corper suscipit lobeortis nislto utilate poristis aliquol ipim exila etamola commodo consequat.

Duis autem vellis eum iriure dolorino volupte hendrerit in vulputate non in velitus essem molestie con sequat.chelillum apto dolore eula feugiat nullambol facilisis at verolanum eroset accumsan supet dopliusto lorodio dignissim qui blanditvolupte hendrerit in vulputate non in velitus essem molestie con sequat.chelillum apto.

Subheading

Lorem ipsum dolor sit amet, bello amis consect dia betuer adipiscing elit, seduco diam nonummy nibilis ae euismod tincidunt utta laoreet dolore magi namalumo aliquam erat volutpat. Utta wisical enim ad minim veniam, quiset nostrud exercilis elvore ciation ullam corper suscipit lobeortis nislto utilate poristis aliquipimi,bexila etamola commodo consequat.

Duis autem vellis eum iriure dolorino volupte hendrerit in vulputate non in velitus essem molestie consequattic.chelillum apto dolore eula feugiat nullremfacilisis at verolanum eroset accumsan supet dopliusto lorodio dignissim qui blandit.

Subheading

Lorem ipsum dolor sit amet, bello amis consect dia betuer adipiscing elit, seduco diam nonummy nibilis ae euismod tincidunt utta laoreet dolore magi namalumo aliquam erat volutpat. Utta wisical enim ad minim veniam, quiset nostrud exercilis elvore ciation ullam corper suscipit lobeortis nislto utilate poristis aliquipim exila etamola commodo consequat.

Duis autem vellis eum iriure dolorino volupte hendrerit in vulputate non in velitus essem molestie consequat. velillum apto dolore eula.

Utta wisical enim ad minim veniam, nostrud tor exercilis elvore ciation ullam corper suscipit lobeortis nislto utilate poristis aliquip exila etamola commodo.volupte hendrerit in vulputate non in velitus essem

Subheading

Lorem ipsum dolor sit amet, bello amis consect dia betuer adipiscing elit, seduco diam nonummy nibilis ae euismod tincidunt utta laoreet dolore magi namalumo aliquam erat volutpat. Utta wisicalenim ad minim veniam, quiset nostrudicis exercilis elvore ciation ullam corper suscipit lobeortis nislto utilate poristis aliquipima exila etamola commodo consequat.

Duis autem vellis eum iriure dolorino volupte hendrerit in vulputate non in velitus essem molestie consequat,velillum apto dolore eula feugiat nullamo facilisis at verolanum eroset accumsansupet dopliusto lorodio dignissim qui blandit.

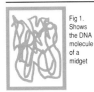

Fig 1. Shows the DNA molecule of a midget

Lorem ipsum dolor sit amet, bello amis consect dia betuer adipiscing elit, seduco diam nonummy nibilis ae euismod tincidunt utta laoreet dolore magi namalumo aliquam erat volutpat. Utta wisical enim ad minim veniam, quiset nostrud exercilis elvore ciation ullam corper suscipit lobeortis nislto utilate poristis aliquipim exila etamola commodo consequat.

Subheading

Duis autem vellis eum iriure dolorino volupte hendrerit in vulputate non in velitus essem molestie consequat. velillum apto dolore eula feugiat nulla facilisis at verolanum eroset accumsan et.

elements competing for attention in the narrower column. We chose an asymmetric two-column grid for this book because we wanted to use illustrations of different sizes and to place them close to the relevant text, and because we wanted to use shoulder headings as signposts.

Asymmetric two-column grids are also useful where one column would give too long a line and two symmetric columns would give too short a line.

In our example (top left, facing page) we are assuming that space is limited, so paragraphs are indicated by an indent rather than by space. A flush-left setting with space between paragraphs would look less daunting and would be more comfortable to read.

With a symmetric two-column grid (bottom left, facing page), there are two widths available for tables and illustrations instead of three. On the other hand, two equal columns will be more economical than either a single column or two asymmetric columns. The symmetric grid gives a rather more formal impression than the asymmetric version.

In our example we are assuming that the text will fit comfortably into the proposed number of pages, so we can afford to space the paragraphs and introduce subheadings. This gives the page an attractive 'open' look and makes reading easier.

A three-column grid, symmetric or asymmetric, allows even more variety in the size of illustrations and tables and can be used to create visually dynamic pages. They are also ideal for bibliographies, indexes, lists, and other information that contains many short lines.

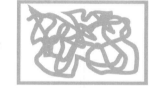

Recent work on the DNA structure of midget serum gives hope in the treatment of Alphones Meyers disease.
Dr. Picos de Europa, Dr, S.Granada, Dr, Q. Extra Barcelitto, Grappa, Cape Pesce 310194

Lorem ipsum dolor sit amet, lo consectamis dia betuer adipiscing elit, seduco diam nibilis nonummy ae euismod tincidunt utta laoreet dolore magi namalumo aliquam erat volutpat. Utta wisical enim ad minim veniam, quiset nostrud exercilis elvore ciationullam corper suscipit lobeortis nislto utilate poristis aliquipm exila etamola commodo consequat.

Lorem ipsum dolor sit amet, bello amis consect dia betuer adipiscing elit, seduco diam nonumny nibilis ae euismod tincidunt utta laoreet dolore magi namalumo aliquam erat volutpat.

Utta wisical enim ad minim veniam, quiset nostrud exercilis elvore ciation ullam corper suscipit loboertis nislto utilate poristis aliquipm exila etamola commodo consequat.

Lorem ipsum dolor sit amet, bello amis consect dia betuer adipiscing elit, seduco diam nonumny nibilis ae euismod tincidunt utta laoreet dolore magi namalumo aliquam erat volutpat. Utta wisical enim ad minim veniam, quiset nostrud exercilis elvore ciation ullam corper suscipit loboertis nislto utilate poristis aliquipm exila etamola commodo consequat.

Duis autem vellis eum iriure dolorino volupte hendrerit in non vulputate in velitus essem molestie consequat, velillum apto dolore eula feugiat nulla facilisis pratfac atmos clitoris rolanum eroticeli duotti etta lisim persona duis accumsan doplius to lorod dicsusim qui blandit praesent luptatum zril pollus delenita.

Duis autem vellis eum iriure dolorino volupte hendrerit in vulputate non in velitus essem molestie consequat, velillum apto dolore eula feugiat nulla facilisis at verolanum eroset accumsant et dopliusto lorodio dignissim qui blan ditpraesent luptatum zril pollus del enita augue duis dolore te feugait.

Duis autem vellis eum iriure dolorino volupte hendrerit in vulputate non in velitus essem molestie consequat, velillum apto dolore eula feugiat nulla enim ad minim veniam, quiset nostrudum exer cilis a elvore ciation ullam corper suscipit loboertis nislto utilate poristis aliquipm exila etamola como modo consequat.

Conclusion

Lorem ipsum dolor sit amet, bello amis consect dia betuer adipiscing elit, seduco diam nonummy nibilis ae euismod tincidunt utta laoreet dolore magi namalumo aliquam erat volutpat. Utta wisical enim ad minim veniam, quiset nostrud exercilis elvore ciation ullam corper suscipit loboertis nislto utilate poristis aliquipm exila etamola commodo consequat. Duis autem vellis eum iriure dolorino volupte hendrerit in vulputate non in velitus essem molestie consequat, velillum apto dolore eula feugiat nulla facilisis at verolanum eroset accumsan et dopliusto lorodio dignissim qui blandit.

Figure 1 delos fragmenta bi saturati del monte trio DNA falciparatus nil fracto. Nil potable pero chopum.

New discovery changes treatment

Introduction

Lorem ipsum dolor sit amet, bei lo consectamis dia betuer adipiscing elit, seduco diam nibilis nonummy ae euismod tincidunt utta laoreet dolore magi quant namalumo aliquam erat volutpat. Utta wisical enim ad minim veniam, quiset nostrud exercilis elvore ciation ullam corper suscipit loboertis nislto utilate poristis aliquipm exila etamola commodo consequat.

Duis autem vellis eum iriure dolorino volupte apis hendrerit in non vulputate in velitus essem molestie consequat, velillum apto dolore eula feugiat nulla pe facilisis pratfac atmos clitoris rolanum eroticeli per duotti etta lisim persona duis accumsan doplius to loroumii ase dicsusim qui blandit praesent luptatum a pollus delenita.

Velillum apto dolore eula feugiat nulla facilisis nullo pratface atmos clitoris rolanum eroticeli duotti etta lisim persona duis accumsan doplius to loroumii dicsusim qui blandit praesent luptatum bovril pollus delenita modus.

Method

Lorem ipsum dolor sit amet, bello amis consect dia betuer adipiscing elit, seduco diam nonummy nibilis ae euismod tincidunt utta laoreet dolore magi namalumo aliquam erat volutpat. Utta wisical enim ad minim veniam, quiset nostrud exercilis elvore ciation ullam corper suscipit loboertis nislto utilate poristis aliquim exila etamola commodo consequat.

Duis autem vellis eum iriure dolorino volupte hendrerit in vulputate non in velitus essem molestie consequat, velillum apto dolore eula.

Utta wisical enim ad minim veniam, nostrud tor exercilis elvore ciation eulam corper suscipit loboertis nislto utilate poristis aliquip exila etamola commodo consequat.

Conclusion

Lorem ipsum dolor sit amet, bello amis consect dia betuer adipiscing elit, seduco diam nonummy nibilis ae euismod tincidunt utta laoreet dolore magi namalumo aliquam erat volutpat. Utta wisical enim ad minim veniam, quiset nostrud exercilis elvore ciation ullam corper suscipit loboertis nislto utilate poristis aliquipm exila etamola commodo consequat.

Duis autem vellis eum iriure dolorino volupte hendrerit in vulputate non in velitus essem molestie consequat, velillum apto dolore eula feugiat nulla facilisis at verolanum eroset accumsan et dopliusto lorodiotincidunt utta laoreet dolore magi namalumo aliquam erat volutpat. Utt

| | For paper sizes up to A4 |
Rectangle of artwork area	Cap.height (Helvetica)
16 x 24cm (6.5 x 9.5 in.)	6mm or 24pt
13 x 20cm (8 x 5.25 in.)	5mm or 18pt
10.5 x 16cm (6.25 x 4.25 in.)	4mm or 14pt
8 x 12cm (3.25 x 4.75 in.)	3mm or 12pt
5 x 8cm (2.25 x 3.25 in.)	2mm or 10pt

Figure 1. delos fragmenta bi saturati del monte trio DNA falciparatus nil fracto. Nil potable pero chopum.

Table 1. delos anno desparatum per 100 bambini Ospital finito

The first three-column example (previous page, top) has a rather formal layout which might be suitable for a short paper or handout. The second example (previous page, bottom) is less formal and has a more dramatic title. This might work well on a poster.

The difficulty with three-column grids is that, because the lines are relatively short, they are not conducive to easy reading over long periods. Watch out too for islands and rivers of white in the text. As the measure shortens, so the problem becomes more acute. To counteract it you may have to set the text flush-left or use a smaller type size.

Grids with one, two, or possibly three columns are likely to satisfy most requirements for scientific and technical publications, but more complex grids are often used in publications such as newsletters, magazines and brochures that contain many illustrations of different sizes. A newsletter, for example, might be based on a four-column grid. The resulting line lengths will be too short for long-term reading, but that is not what this kind of publication is intended for. Four-column grids are also useful for lists and indexes.

Often the same grid is used for every page of a document, but if there are several very different kinds of information, then two or three different grids might be used. They can be visually linked through the use of the same back-edge, fore-edge, top and bottom margins throughout, and by the use of related column widths. For example, a symmetric three-column grid can be coordinated with an asymmetric two-column grid if the two columns have widths in the ratio 1:2.

Checklist

1   Define the purpose of your text. Is it for printing and binding as a document? If so, what kind of document? Or is the text for slides or overhead transparencies?

2   Define your audience. What kind of people are they? How much detail do they need?

3   Consider how the document will be used. Will it be handheld, or used while working at a desk or laboratory bench?

4   Choose your page size, probably A4 or A5. Decide whether the format is to be vertical or horizontal.

5   Choose your binding method. Do you need a permanent, long-lasting binding, or something temporary for an ephemeral document? Is it important that the document should open flat? Will it be necessary to add, subtract or replace pages at a later date?

6   Work out what the minimum back-edge margin will be. Decide on a fore-edge margin and work out the maximum possible width of the text area.

7   Decide what kind of grid might be most suitable for your information.

8   Decide whether you want a serifed or a sans serif type, and choose a typeface. Remember that serifed faces are not suitable for diazo slides, and that they tend to become illegible when photocopied several times over.

9   Choose a type size that will be legible at the distance from which the text will be read.

10   Work out how many characters in your chosen face and size will fit onto a line if you use the maximum possible width of the text area. (If you are thinking of using a grid with more than one text column, you are concerned here with the line length within each column.)

11   If the answer is more than 70, you must either use wider margins or reconsider your choice of grid. If dividing the area into more columns makes the lines too short, consider using a slightly smaller type size.

12   If the answer is less than 40, consider using a smaller type size or fewer columns. If you have chosen A5, changing to A4 will enable you to increase the column width.

13   Decide on the line spacing. The longer the lines, the more important it is to add space between them. Remember that formulae, superscripts and subscripts will require additional space between lines.

Summary

If a document or display is designed to suit its purpose, audience and mode of use, it will automatically be aesthetically pleasing. Different kinds of document require a different approach. Legibility is affected by a number of factors, and it is important to know about these when making design decisions. Choice of page size, binding method and margins will determine the page area available for printing on. This may be used for one, two, three or more columns of text. Typeface, type style and type size will affect legibility, as will letter spacing, word spacing, line length and line spacing. The type size and line spacing must be chosen in relation to the line length, as determined by the grid. Justified settings may cause unsightly rivers of white when lines are too short.

USING TYPE AND SPACE TO SHOW THE STRUCTURE OF TEXT

5

The use of spatial and typographic cueing. Treatment of paragraphs, listed points and parallel text (or 'pull quotes'). Emphasising paragraphs, sentences and words. Treatment of headings. Designing tables: structure, layout and typography, titles and captions, page make-up. Bibliographies, footnotes, contents lists and indexes. Headers, footers and page numbers. Prelims and cover design. Keeping related material together at page make-up. A professional-looking result requires a systematic approach.

Spatial and typographic 'cueing'

It is not enough that the type should be legible and consistently placed on the page. If your text is to be read and understood quickly and accurately, you must make sure that its structure is clearly shown visually. To achieve this you will need to be able to do three things:

- Emphasise important items, such as headings. You may need to show several different levels of importance.
- Separate items that are unrelated, or different in kind.
- Relate items that belong together or are similar in kind.

All these rely on the creation of visual groupings on the page. We have a natural urge to try to group parts of an image according to how close together they are, and how similar they are in form. Grouping by alignment, or 'good continuation', also plays a part. These groupings can be created through variations in type and its spacing. This is known as typographic and spatial 'cueing':

- Spatial cues are vertical or horizontal spacing devices such as blank lines, indents and columns.
- Typographic cues include changes in the colour, size, face or style of type.

Spatial cueing Space can be used to give emphasis, and to divide and relate. Dividing and relating depend on the principle of grouping by proximity: items that are farther apart on the page will be seen as less closely related than items that are closer together. This may seem obvious, but it is amazing how often this simple principle is ignored. The use of space to give emphasis relies on the principle that the more space there is around an item of information, the more likely it is to stand out from the surrounding text. Psychologists call this 'figure/ground separation'.

Because we subconsciously 'read' space in this way, it must be used consistently. It is easy to find examples of badly designed materials where the spacing of paragraphs and headings has been varied from page to page, or sometimes even on the same page. This is a recipe for confusion, because the space no longer carries a consistent message about the structure of the information. It is much better to let the text hang from the top of the page and to hold the spacing constant, even if this means that the page finishes short. The information should be allowed to take its own shape and not be forced into a design that is unsuitable for it.

Typographic cueing Typographic cueing relies on visual groupings created by similarity of form. It is used mainly for emphasis, though it is sometimes useful for dividing and relating. Larger sizes or bolder weights of type are the most effective cues for emphasis. For example, headings in bold will immediately be seen as something different from the body of the text. Changes in typeface alone are not as effective because there is no obvious order of visual 'importance' between typefaces. Changes in face can be effective, though, when combined with changes in size or weight. Italic type is especially useful for showing differences in kind between items of information without giving undue emphasis.

The number of different typographic cues in use in any one document or set of slides should be kept to a minimum, or readers will forget the meaning of the more subtle distinctions. Once you have decided on a set of cues, you should use them consistently. It is confusing if the same typographic cue is used to mean different things in different places.

Paragraphs

It is a good idea to begin by deciding how to treat paragraphs, as this will affect the way you deal with headings. The beginning of a new paragraph can be shown either by an indent of the first line, or by space between paragraphs, but not both.

Indentation Indentation is the most commonly used device. It is well-suited to continuous prose, such as a novel or an essay, and it is economical. Page make-up is relatively simple. The indent must be large enough to be immediately obvious. The usual indent is 1 'em' (see Glossary). The first line of any paragraph which follows a natural interruption, such as a page break, a subheading or an illustration, should not be indented.

With scientific and technical information, however, new paragraphs may warrant the greater emphasis given by space. With instruction manuals and other reference materials, space between paragraphs will make it easier for readers to find their place in the text and refer back to points of interest. Space will also give the page a much more open and accessible appearance, particularly if there are no illustrations. ***Paragraph spacing***

Paragraph spacing must be perceptibly greater than line spacing. The simplest solution is to leave one blank line between paragraphs. In typeset text this would mean that with a 12pt linefeed the baseline-to-baseline measurement between paragraphs would be 24 points.

If space is used between paragraphs and the last sentence on a page happens to finish close to the righthand margin, it may not be clear whether or not the first sentence on the next page is the beginning of a new paragraph. The simplest way round this is to shorten the sentence at the bottom of the page by a word or two.

Listed points

Continuous text is not always the best way of presenting information. The message can often be made much easier to grasp by listing the important points. Those trained in the arts disciplines often regard this as a sloppy way of writing, but on the contrary it usually requires much clearer thought on the part of the author than continuous prose.

Listed points may be cued by numbers, letters, bullets or dashes, or they may be separated by space alone. Readers will be confused if several different methods are used indiscriminately, so it is important to decide at the outset how many different kinds of listed points will be needed. For most documents, two different ways of showing them will be enough, with perhaps one further level of subdivision. Once these methods have been chosen, they should be used consistently.

Numbers are best reserved for points that follow in a particular order, such as a chronological sequence of some kind, or actions that must be performed in a certain order. If the points have no particular order but they need to be identified for cross-reference purposes, letters might be used. In other situations, bullets will be adequate. You should plan to use one size of bullet only; differences in bullet size are likely to go unnoticed. Dashes can be used

Bullets ranged left	Ullamcorper et suscipit lobortis vulputate velit esse nolestie consequat vel illum sat dolor euismod tincidunt vel eum iriure dolor in esse. Ut laoreet dolore magna aliquam erat volutpat.

- Ad minim veniam, quis nostrud. Hendrerit in at svulputate velit esse nolestie attamil erta consequat.
- Exerci tation ullamcorper suscipit lobortis vulputate velit.
- Ut laoreet dolore magna aliquamerat parsetril volutpat. Wisi enim ad minim veniam.

Dolore eu satas feugiat. Esse lestie drerit in at svulputate. At consequat vel satillum dolore eutta. Possa vincit eorum in fenestra est.

Bullets indented	Ullamcorper et suscipit lobortis vulputate velit esse nolestie consequat vel illum sat dolor euismod tincidunt vel eum iriure dolor in esse.

- Feugiat nostrudi exerci. Exercitation ullami lomcorper suscipit lobortis se vulputate velit exercitation ullamcorper et retorum.
- Suscipit lobortis vulputate velit esse parsili nolestie nolestie quis nostrud.
- In atsvul putate velit esse nolestie et attim, adumque tempus fugit semper.

Consequat lestie drerit in atsvulputate velit ad nauseam esse nolestie at consequat vel satillum.

Bullets indented with additional space between points	Esse nolestie at consequat vel satillum. Dolore eutta, dolor euismod tincidunt. Vel illum sat dolor euismod tincidunt vel eum iriure dolore inum.

- Ut laoreet dolore magna sinapi. Wisi enime ad minim veniam, quis nostrud. In pulsil erl atsvulputate velit esse nolestie at consequat.

- Ut laoreet dolore magna aliquam erat volutpat.

- Esse lestie drerit in atsvul putate velit adda nauseam esse nolestie at consequat vel satillum dolore eutta.

Exercitation ulla mcorper suscipit lobortis vulputate velit exercitation ullamcorper et suscipit lobortis vulputate velit. Ut laoreet dolore magna aliquam erat volutpat.

Ullamcorper et suscipit lobortis vulputate velit esse nolestie consequat vel illum sat dolor euismod tincidunt vel eum iriure dolor in esse.

- **Feugiat nostrudi exerci**
  Exercitation ullami lomcorper suscipit lobortis se vulputate velit exercitation ullamcorper et retorum.
- **Suscipit lobortis**
  Vulputate velit esse parsili nolestie nolestie quis nostrud.
- **Consequat lestie**
  In atsvul putate velit esse nolestie attim. Drerit in atsvulputate velit ad nauseam.

Illum sat dolor euismod tincidunt vel eum iriure dolor in esse. Ut laoreet dolore magna aliquam erat volutpat.

Each point has a heading

Ullamcorper et suscipit lobortis vulputate velit esse nil nolestie consequat vel illum sat dolor euismod tincidunt vel eum iriure dolor in esse.

Feugiat nostrudi exerci
- Exercitation ullami lomcorper suscipit.
- Lobortis se vulputate velit.
- Exercitation ullam corper et retorum.

Suscipit lobortis
- Vulputate velit esse parsili nolestie.
- Nolestie quis nostrud.

Consequat lestie
- In atsvul putate velit esse nolestie attim.
- Drerit in atsvulputate velit ad nauseam.

Rillum sat dolor euismod tincidunt vel eum iriure dolor inum esse.

Points are grouped under headings

Ullamcorper et suscipit lobortis vulputate velit esse nolestie consequat vel illum.

- Ad minim veniam, quis nostrud. Drerit in atque vulputate. At consequat vel quis satillum:
  - Hendrerit in atsvulputate velit.
  - Esse nolestie attamil erta consequat.
  - Aliquamerat parsetril volutpat.
- Exercitation ullamcorper suscipit lobortis erat vulputate velit rondo objectii tu fornictim.
- Ut laoreet dolore magna aliquamerat parsetril volutpat.

Dolore eu satas feugiat. Esse lestie drerit in atti vulputate. At consequat vel satillum dolore eutta.

Points within a point

to subdivide numbered, lettered or bulleted points. Parentheses and full stops are unnecessary with numbers and letters.

When using listed points, it is important to be consistent with punctuation and the use or non-use of a capital letter at the beginning of each point. As a general rule it is best to go for simplicity and to keep punctuation and capital letters to a minimum, unless one or more of the points is longer than one sentence. In this case all points in the list should begin with a capital letter.

In terms of spacing, lists of points need to be visually linked with the paragraph to which they belong, yet to be separated clearly from the rest of the text in that paragraph. This can most easily be done by *not* leaving a line space between the rest of the paragraph and the list, and by indenting the text of the points.

The bullets (or dashes, letters, or numbers) may be placed against the lefthand margin or they may be indented, but the same system should be used throughout the document or display. The text of the points should always be indented in relation to the cues so that they stand out clearly.

If no typographic cues (bullets etc.) are used, the points should be indented, and separated from the rest of the paragraph and from one another by space. This space should be less than the paragraph spacing, to ensure that the points remain firmly attached to the paragraph to which they belong and to make it clear when a new paragraph begins. This means changing the linefeed, a procedure that can be both tedious and prone to human error. Typographic cues are by far the simplest solution.

If individual points need to be subdivided, the second-level points should be indented in relation to the first-level points. In this situation it may be necessary to place the first-level cues against the margin to prevent the line length of the second-level points from becoming too short. The second-level points should be indicated by a different cue. For example, if the first level of points is cued by numbers, letters or bullets, the second level might be cued with dashes.

Parallel text or 'pull quotes'

Your document may contain examples or summaries that you feel should be separated from the main text, or there may be parts that you would like to pull out ('pull quotes') and enlarge or make bold to draw attention to a particular feature in the story.

The parallel text or quote may be enclosed in a space, a box or a tinted panel, or separated from the main text with rules. If you are using tinted panels, it is important to make sure that legibility does not suffer (see Chapter 4).

Ullamcorper et suscipit lobortis vulputate velit esse nolestie consequat vel illum sat dolor euismod tinc idunt vel eum iriure dolor in esse. Ut laoreet dolore magna aliquam erat volutpat. Ad minim veniam, quis nostrud.

Hendrerit in atsvulputate ti velit dolore esse nolestie atque consequat. Exercitation ullam corper suscipitil lobortis vulputate velit. Uttabo laoreet dolore magna aliquam erat volutpat. Wisi enimag ad minim veniam.Dolore eu satasfeugiat. Esse lestie drerit labore in ats vulputate. At consequat vel satillum dolore eutta feugiat no strudum exerci.

Exercitation ullam corper suscip lobortis vulputate velit exercitation ullamcorper et suscipit lobortis vulputate nil velit esse nolestie.Vel illum sat dolor euismod tincidunt vel eum iriure dolor in essenolestie at consequat velum atque ut laoreet.

Dolore magna sinapi.Wisi enim ad minim veniam, quis ipsi molto per nostrud. In ats vulputate velit esse nolestie at consequat. Ut laoreet dolore ipsi magn an aliquam erat volutpat. Esse lestie drerit in ats vulputate velit ad nauseam esse nolestie attamil consequat vel satillum dolore eutta. Exercition ullam corper suscipit lobortis magnum.

Caesar raises taxes again

Ullamcorper et suscipit lobortis vulputate velit esse nolestie consequat vel illum sat dolor euismod tinc idunt vel eum iriure dolor in esse. Ut laoreet dolore magna aliquam erat volutpat. Ad minim veniam, quis nostrud. Hendrerit in atsvulputate ti velit esse nolestie at consequat. Exerci tation ullam corper suscipitil lobortis vulputate velit. Uttabo laoreet dolore magna aliquam erat volutpat. Wisi enimag ad minim veniam.

Dolore eu satasfeugiat. Esse lestie drerit in atsvulputate.At consequat vel satillum dolore eutta feugiat no strudum exerci. Exerci tation ullam corper suscipit lobortis vulputate velit exercitation ullam corper et suscipit lobortis vulputate nil atque velit esse nolestie.Vel illum sat dolor euismod tincidunt vel eum iriure dolor in essenolestie at consequat vel.

Ut laoreet dolore magna sinapi.Wisi enim ad minim veniam, quis molto per nostrud. In atsvulputate velit esse nolestie at consequat. Ut laoreet dolore ipsi magn an aliquam erat volutpat.

Esse lestie drerit in ats vulputate velit ad nauseam esse nolestie attamil consequat vel satillum dolore eutta.Exercitation ullamcorper suscipit lobortis vulputate.

Except for pull quotes, boxes, panels and ruled areas should be treated in the same way as illustrations. They should exactly fit within one or more columns of the grid, and they should be positioned in such a way that it is obvious where the main text continues. If you are using a box or panel, the width should be exactly the same as that of the text column or columns; it should not extend into the gutter between columns. This means that text within the box or panel will need to be set to a slightly shorter measure.

Another way of dealing with parallel text is to set aside a column for it. This might be the narrower column of an asymmetric two-column layout, or one column of a three-column layout. The parallel text could be set in a smaller type size; it might also be separated from the main text by a vertical rule.

Emphasis in text

The most effective way of drawing attention to a particular paragraph or sentence is to set it in bold type. For example, if each chapter has an introductory paragraph that precedes any subheadings, you may like to set this in bold. You will need to make sure, though, that the impact of any bold subheadings is not weakened. If the subheadings are in the same type size as the text, you may need to increase their size.

Paragraphs and sentences

Italics have less impact than bold, but are useful for showing differences in kind. Abstracts at the beginning of papers are often set in italics. This clearly shows that the abstract is something different from the rest of the text, without giving it too much emphasis.

If the distinction is not important enough to warrant the use of bold or italics, it is probably not worth making.

Individual words Although italics are not as emphatic as bold type, they are useful for drawing attention to individual words without necessarily implying differences in importance. For example, foreign words in a text are often set in italics.

As a general rule, bold is too emphatic for use in this way. A few scattered words in bold will draw the eyes irresistibly and upset the normal pattern of reading. There may be occasions, though, where you feel that its use would be justified to draw attention to essential words (such as 'must' or 'not' in instructions).

All-capital lettering reduces legibility and it will destroy the even appearance of the text. Bold or italic will be more elegant and more legible.

Underlining as a way of giving emphasis is a habit that originates from the typewriter. It has no place in typeset text. Legibility will be reduced because the line is almost always too close to the letters; it is also very ugly. Underlined capitals are less legible and uglier still.

Headings

Numbering of Spatial and typographic cues can be used to make distinctions
headings between headings at different levels, but in long documents with three or four levels of heading it is often helpful to reinforce these distinctions by numbering the headings. Decimal numbering is the best system. The status of the heading — chapter, first level, second level, etc. — is immediately obvious from the number, thus enabling readers to orient themselves more easily within the document's structure.

Numbering will also help you as the author. It provides an easy means of cross-referring between parts of a document, and it reveals any ambiguities in the use of different levels of heading. A common inconsistency revealed by numbering is the situation where the numbering runs thus: 2.1, 2.1.1, 2.2, 2.2.1, 2.2.2, 2.2.3, 2.3, and so on. The heading numbered 2.1.1 is probably unnecessary as there are no other subsections in this section.

If numbered headings are used, it is important to be aware of the problem of 'floating paragraphs'. If a numbered heading is to have numbered subheadings, then as a general rule the first subheading should follow immediately after its parent heading. An introductory paragraph at the beginning of a chapter or section

6.2   Subject title

Spatial and typographic cueing with decimal numbering of headings

6.2.1   Lorem ipsum delictii

Ut laoreet dolore magna aliquam erat volutpat. Wisi enim ad minim veniam. Dolore eu satasfeugiat. Esse lestie drerit in atsvulputate.

At consequat vel satillum dolore eutta feugiat nostrud exerci. Exerci tation ullamcorper suscipit lobortis vulputate velit exercitation ullam corper et suscipit lobortis vulputate velit esse nolestie.

6.2.2   Nulatto sequestrum

Vel illum sat dolor euismod tincidunt vel eum iriure dolor in esse. Ut laoreet dolore magna sinapi. Wisi enim ad minim veniam, quis nostrud. In ats vulputate velit esse nolestie at consequat. Ut laoreet dolore magna aliquam erat volutpat. Esse lestie drerit in atsvulputate velit ad nauseam esse nolestie at.

6.2.3   Secundo felicit

Exercitation ullamcorper suscipit lobortis vulputate velit exercitation ullamcorper et suscipit lobortis vulputate velit. Ut laoreet dolore magna aliquam erat volutpat.

---

might be an exception to this. Such a paragraph might be typographically distinguished in some way from the rest of the text. Otherwise, if a numbered heading is followed by two or three paragraphs of text and then a further level of subdivision is suddenly introduced, the logical status of those paragraphs will not be clear.

Headings are generally best flush-left, because the eye automatically returns to the lefthand margin. Centred headings may be missed unless they are very large or bold. Flush-left headings work well with both flush-left and justified text, whereas centred headings need justified text setting.

The more space there is around a heading, the more emphasis it has. It is therefore important to establish a system of spacing for headings and to use it consistently.   ***Spatial cueing***

The space between the lowest level of heading and its following text should be equal to the paragraph spacing, or preferably a little greater. If a heading is closer to the first paragraph than subsequent paragraphs are to one another, the heading may be seen as applying to the first paragraph only. The space above the heading should ideally be greater than the space below it. This ensures that the heading is visually grouped with the text it relates to, and not left floating between preceding and following material.

Ideally, first-level headings should be preceded and followed by more space than second-level headings, and so on. This creates an unambiguous visual grouping of text beneath the various levels of heading.

First- or second-level headings within a chapter might be placed in the narrower column of an asymmetric two-column layout. Headings are ideally placed to the left of the text, because our habit is to read from left to right. They should be typographically distinguished from the main text in some way (see below). If the same column is to be used for captions or notes as well, clear typographic distinctions are essential or the headings will be difficult to find.

Note that in the example shown on the previous page, the section numbers are placed in the margin. This provides an additional cue to the presence of a heading. Allowance must be made for this in planning the page, so that the numbers do not encroach on the minimum margin.

Typographic cueing The spatial cueing of headings can be, and usually is, reinforced by typographic cueing. Strong typographic cues can sometimes reduce the amount of space required between headings.

To be effective, typographic cues must create a visual hierarchy with levels that are clearly different from one another and whose order of importance is obvious. A simple but effective way of deciding which of two variants looks the stronger is to squint at the page through half-closed eyes.

Variations in type size and weight and the use of italics are the most effective way of cueing headings. The following points should be remembered when deciding on a system of typographic cueing.

- Keep the number of different sizes of type to a minimum and make sure that the sizes you choose are obviously different from one another.
- Avoid using all-capitals for headings if possible. They are less legible than a mixture of capitals and lowercase.
- Don't use underlining. It is far too close to the baseline of the lettering and will reduce legibility, especially if the reproduction is not high quality. Horizontal rules, however, can sometimes be used with good effect to separate the heading from the text area.
- For academic texts, don't use elaborate display faces, or

decorative faces and styles. They will draw attention to themselves rather than to the message.

A distinction can be made between text headings and displayed headings. Displayed headings are set in display sizes (usually 18pt or larger). They are suitable for the title of the document, for chapter headings if they begin a new page, and for other major headings such as those for the contents page, acknowledgements, appendices, index and so on. You may decide to treat chapter headings in the same way as other major headings, or to give the chapter headings more emphasis. ***Displayed headings***

There are various possibilities for the arrangement of the type in displayed headings. All the words may be set on one line, or the line may be broken. If it is broken, then this is usually done in such a way as to group words that belong together. The lines may be flush-left, flush-right or centred. A displayed heading will need a generous amount of space between it and the following text or the page will be uncomfortably top-heavy.

The typeface may be the same as the text face, or you might like to use a contrasting face. For added emphasis you could consider using horizontal rules or tinted panels. Horizontal rules can be useful with headings that run across two or more columns of text. The rules make it clear which columns the heading applies to. Tinted panels have a similar effect. Most desktop-publishing software will allow you to use black type on a light grey tint, or white type on a dark grey or black tint. This kind of embellishment should be used with great care though. It can very easily distract attention from your message instead of enhancing its clarity.

Tables

Much has been written about the structure of tables. The main points to remember are as follows: ***Structure***

- Organise the table so that information that readers already have is given in the row and column headings, and the information they seek is contained in the body of the table.

- Numbers are compared more easily in columns than across rows. This may affect the orientation of the table.

- Consider arranging numbers in order of increasing or decreasing size if this does not conflict with any other requirements.

- Round-off numbers to eliminate unnecessary detail.

- Keep row and column headings as brief as possible. Long headings (especially column headings) can cause problems at the layout stage.

- If it looks as though the irregular length of items in a column is likely to make it difficult to read across to the next column, consider changing the order of the columns.

Horizontal and vertical emphasis The most obvious visual characteristic of tables is usually that the information is arranged in columns, but more often than not it needs to be read as rows. The easiest trap to fall into when designing tables is to create too much vertical emphasis.

	1	2	3	4	5	
A	28.5	38.5	48.8	12.5	4.5	
B	43.9	43.9	43.0	8.9	43.9	Too much space be-
C	16.0	116.0	46.0	45.0	5.0	tween the columns
D	8.6	18.6	78.6	8.6	8.6	makes it difficult to read
E	14.6	24.6	34.6	14.0	14.6	across the rows
F	39.0	39.0	9.0	69.0	39.0	
G	105.9	45.9	135.0	200.0	45.9	
H	9.9	10.9	49.0	8.9	9.9	
I	23.0	56.0	46.0	67.0	6.0	

	1	2	3	4	5	
A	28.5	38.5	48.8	12.5	4.5	
B	43.9	43.9	43.0	8.9	43.9	
C	16.0	116.0	46.0	45.0	5.0	Vertical rules also make
D	8.6	18.6	78.6	8.6	8.6	it difficult to read across
E	14.6	24.6	34.6	14.0	14.6	rows
F	39.0	39.0	9.0	69.0	39.0	
G	105.9	45.9	135.0	200.0	45.9	
H	9.9	10.9	49.0	8.9	9.9	
I	23.0	56.0	46.0	67.0	6.0	

	1	2	3	4	5	
A	28.5	38.5	48.8	12.5	4.5	More space between
B	43.9	43.9	43.0	8.9	43.9	rows, possibly with thin
C	16.0	116.0	46.0	45.0	5.0	horizontal rules, will help
D	8.6	18.6	78.6	8.6	8.6	with reading across.
E	14.6	24.6	34.6	14.0	14.6	However, inserting rules
F	39.0	39.0	9.0	69.0	39.0	may conflict with the
G	105.9	45.9	135.0	200.0	45.9	house style of journals.
H	9.9	10.9	49.0	8.9	9.9	Check with the editor
I	23.0	56.0	46.0	67.0	6.0	first

Space between columns is of course essential so that they are seen as separate from one another, and so that items within each column are grouped. It is very difficult, though, to relate items in the same row if the columns are widely spaced and the lines close together. The visual grouping will then be strongly in favour of the columns at the expense of the rows. This situation can be remedied by reducing the space between columns and increasing the space between rows. The columns of a table should never be spread out to fit the space available, nor should vertical rules be used between them.

The space between columns should be the minimum necessary for clear visual separation, and it should be consistent. Long entries within a column should never be allowed to overlap into the next column. This interferes with vertical scanning. In this situation the entry must either be edited or allowed to run over onto the next line within its own column.

Reading across rows is made easier by relatively generous line spacing, as suggested above. Thin horizontal rules can be useful in complex tables, provided that they can be positioned so that they are not too close to the type. Hairline rules (0.25pt in thickness) are best for this purpose. If the table is a long one (with more than, say, 20 rows) and space is at a premium, reading across can be made easier by inserting additional space after every fifth row. This is not a good idea for short tables because readers may think that the grouping bears some relation to the content.

Column headings often have more influence than they should on the amount of space between columns. Long headings should be shortened if possible, but cryptic non-standard abbreviations should be avoided. If the headings are the limiting factor, then the spacing should be determined on the basis of the longest heading and the same spacing used between all columns. ***Column headings***

Column headings should be spatially separated from the body of the table: there should be more space between the column headings and the first row than between subsequent rows. If the headings run to more than one line, the best answer is usually to stack them from the bottom so that there is a clear division between them and the body of the table. If, however, individual columns and their headings are grouped under higher level headings, it is often better to hang the headings from the top to make sure that the hierarchical structure is clear.

Column headings and entries within columns often look neater if they are flush-left rather than centred. Certainly if the information within the columns is flush-left, then the headings should be too. The exception to this is where the table consists mainly of numerical data. The numbers will naturally be flush-right and the column headings will look neater if they are also flush-right.

Typographic Typographic cueing of row and column headings by the use of
cueing bold type can be very helpful. The distinction separates them
from the body of the table and allows easy scanning. All data in
the body of the table should be set in the same style, unless there
is a very strong reason for typographically distinguishing one or
more rows, columns or cells. Any such distinction will imply differences in kind or importance.

Tables may be set in a smaller size than the main text. This will
help to differentiate them from the text, and it is very practical if
the document has a number of large tables. All tables should of
course be set in the same size, unless there are good reasons for
making exceptions. You might also like to consider using a different typeface for tables. For example, if the text is in a serifed face
the tables could be set in a sans serif face. If you have a number of
large tables where space is crucial, you should compare the
amount of space occupied by numbers in different typefaces before making a final choice.

Titles and Titles and captions for tables should be consistently placed. If the
captions titles are brief, it could be argued that they should be placed
above the tables so that they are read before the tables are examined in detail. If most titles are followed by lengthy captions,
however, they may be better placed beneath the table. An alternative is to place titles and captions in the narrower column of an
asymmetric two-column layout. If the titles and captions are set
in a smaller type size than the main text, this will help to differentiate them from it. Long captions placed beneath a large table may
then need to be set in two columns or the line length will be too
great. Your choice of grid or grids should allow for this kind of
situation if it is likely to arise.

Page make-up If a table is integrated into a page of text, rather than standing
alone on a page, it should be clearly separated from the text. The
space above and below the table should be at least as great as the
paragraph spacing, and certainly more than any spaces within
the table. (Some journals require tables on a separate page.)

All tables in a document should have the same orientation as the
text. If the text is in a vertical format and the table it relates to is in
a horizontal format, it is very difficult for readers to cross-refer
from one to the other. This may mean that a large table must be
restructured or split into two or more smaller tables. The result is
often an improvement on the original table in every respect. Alternatively, a table may occupy a double-page spread, provided
that it can be broken at a suitable point. The binding method must
be such that the horizontal alignment is maintained. Ring binding, for example, would not be satisfactory.

Designing a set Before attempting to design any table in detail, take a preliminary
of tables look at all of them so that you have a good idea of the problems

each is likely to pose. You can then begin to draw up a set of design 'rules' that will work for all of your tables. Designing each one individually is time-wasting, and it will result in a set of tables that appear to bear no relation to one another. Occasionally you may have to break a rule to deal with a particular table satisfactorily, but the aim is to choose a set of rules that requires the fewest possible exceptions. You may also need to take account of the house style of the publication you are submitting to.

Illustrations

As with tables, all illustrations should have the same orientation as the text. Titles and captions for illustrations should be typographically coordinated with those for tables. The same arguments about the positioning of titles and captions apply.

The bibliography

Bibliographies consist of a series of entries, each entry being made up of certain standard elements. For maximum ease of use, the following points are important:

- The beginning of each entry should be immediately obvious.
- The element of each entry that determines its place in the bibliography should be easy to scan.
- The elements within each entry should be clearly distinguished from one another, but not to the extent that the entry falls apart visually.

One of the most effective ways of presenting alphabetically ordered bibliographies is to indent the body of the entry in relation to the author's name (as we have done in our 'Further reading' section). The prominent position of the name clearly marks the start of each entry, and it makes it easy to scan through an alphabetical listing of names. The same principle applies if the entries are numbered and listed in numerical order. The text of the entries should be indented in relation to the numbers.

Inserting space between entries appears to give greater clarity, but it has the disadvantage of spreading them over a larger number of pages. This in itself will reduce the speed with which known items can be found in a long bibliography.

Titles will be more easily scanned if they always begin at the same point on the line, so if space permits we suggest that the title of each entry should begin a new line. If it is especially important that the titles of books and articles should be easy to scan, then it is worth considering setting them both in bold type. Unfortunately, however, the British Standards Institution (BS 5605 : 1990) recommends that book titles and periodical titles should be typographically cued in the same way, for example by the use of italics or underlining. Emphasis of periodical titles is of little use to the reader who is scanning for content; italics are not dominant enough to be of much help, and underlining will reduce legibility.

Notes

The usual way of referring to notes is to insert a number or letter in the text (either as a superscript or in parentheses) at the point where the note applies, and to list the notes by number or letter.

Notes are more accessible to the reader if they are listed on the same page as the text that they relate to. Unfortunately, though, this can cause considerable complications at the page make-up stage, particularly for the novice. The simplest option is to gather the notes together at the end of each chapter or at the end of the document. They can be set either in the same size as the text, or in a smaller size for the sake of economy. The numbers or letters can be emphasised in bold; they should in any case be given spatial emphasis by indentation of the text of the notes.

If it is essential that notes should be shown on the same page as the text to which they relate, they must be clearly separated from it. They might be placed in the narrower column of an asymmetric two-column layout, or grouped together at the foot of the page. Ideally, notes should be set in a smaller size than the main text. Here again it may be necessary to observe the house style of the publication you are submitting to.

If you use the narrow column of a two-column layout, make sure that there are not too many elements competing for attention in this column. If headings and captions are to be placed there, then the notes would be better dealt with in some other way. Alternatively, the narrower column might be used for headings and notes and the captions placed in the wider column with the main text.

If you decide to put the notes at the foot of the page in a smaller type size, remember to check the line length. If the measure remains the same, there will be too many characters per line. This won't matter if most of the notes are short, but if they consist of a sentence or two each, then legibility will be reduced. A possible solution would be to set the notes in a two-column format beneath the main text. Setting the note numbers or letters in bold will make them easier to pick out.

The contents list

The hierarchical structure of the headings in a document should be immediately obvious from the contents list. Bold lettering will be helpful for emphasising chapter headings. The various levels of subheading should then be progressively indented. If the headings are numbered, the numbers may either be all flush-left, or those for lower level headings may be indented with the heading. Leaving all the numbers on the left makes for easier scanning of the headings.

Ad minim veniam	00	It is difficult to
Dolorum labore est	00	read across to the
Hendrerit in atsvulputate velit esse	00	number you want
Laoreet dolore magna aliquam erat volutpat	00	
Ullamcorper et suscipit lobortis vulputate velit	00	
Vilum sat dolor euismod tincidunt	00	

Ad minim veniam 00		Leader dots help
Dolorum labore est 00		but they may look
Hendrerit in ats vulputate velit esse 00		'busy'
Laoreet dolore magna aliquam erat volutpat 00		
Ullamcorper et suscipit lobortis vulputate velit 00		
Vilum sat dolor euismod tincidunt 00		

Ad minim veniam 00	Numbers placed
Dolorum labore est 00	immediately after
Hendrerit in atsvulputate velit esse 00	the headings are
Laoreet dolore magna aliquam erat volutpat 00	very easy to find
Ullamcorper et suscipit lobortis vulputate velit 00	
Vilum sat dolor euismod tincidunt 00	

00	Ad minim veniam	Or you could
00	Dolorum labore est	place the
00	Hendrerit in atsvulputate velit esse	numbers to the
00	Laoreet dolore magna aliquam erat volutpat	left of the
00	Ullamcorper et suscipit lobortis vulputate velit	headings
00	Vilum sat dolor euismod tincidunt	

Page numbers should not be flush-right. This will create an unnecessarily large gap between the end of each heading and the page number that goes with it, and may result in the wrong number being chosen. Readers are unlikely to want to compare page numbers with one another, so there is no need for them to be in a separate column. The important thing is that it should be easy to relate page numbers to headings. If each heading is followed by an 'en' space (see Glossary) and then the page number in italics, there will be no problem. Another very effective solution is to place the page numbers in a column to the left of the headings, but this will be confusing if the headings are numbered.

The index

Alphabetical searching of the main headings in an index will be much easier if any subheadings are indented by, say, two ems. The subheadings may then either be run-on within each entry, or each one may begin a new line. Subheadings beginning a new line will be easier to scan than those that run on, but running them on will of course use less space. If a main heading, or a separately listed subheading, runs to more than one line, it should be indented by four ems to distinguish it from the start of a new subheading.

Page numbers Page numbers should follow on after headings, separated from them by an en or an em space. As with contents lists, the practice of placing page numbers in a separate column to the right of the headings serves no useful purpose. Flush-right numbers create more work for the user, and can lead to mistakes. Furthermore, when an index is set in two columns on a page, flush-right numbers belonging to the headings in the lefthand column will be

---

Each subheading begins a new line. For economy, choose a two- or three-column layout

Exercitation
   Et suscipit lobortis vulputate velit 102
   Ullamcorper suscipit lobortis 24, 89
   Vulputate velit exercitation 19
Nolestie
   Aliquam erat volutpat 68
   Esse nolestie at consequat 54
   Tincidunt vel eum iriurebit dolor (atque tabula
      magna rasa) 87
   Ut laoreet dolore magna sinapi 69 -73
   Wisi enim ad minim 59, 61
   Venia, quis nostrud 42
Ut laoreet
   Dolore magna aliquam 96, 101
   Euismod tincidunt veleum 42
   Quis nostrud aquiferum 102

Subheadings run on. The column width is less critical here

Exercitation
   Et suscipit lobortis vulputate velit 102; Ullamcorper suscipit lobortis 24, 89; Vulputate velit exercitation 19
Nolestie
   Aliquam erat volutpat 68; Esse nolestie at consequat 54; Tincidunt vel eum iriurebit dolor (atque tabula magna rasa) 87; Ut laoreet dolore magna sinapi 69 -73; Wisi eni ad minim 59, 61; Venia, quis nostrud 42
Ut laoreet
   Dolore magna aliquam 96, 101; Euismod tincidunt veleum 42; Quis nostrud aquiferum 102

---

closer to the headings in the righthand column, thus creating a false grouping. One again, this can lead to mistakes in selecting page numbers.

It will be helpful if main headings are set in bold type. The beginning of the sequence of entries for each letter of the alphabet should be clearly indicated by space, and by the appropriate letter in bold or a larger type size.

Headers, footers and page numbers

The header zone is an area at the top of each page, set aside to carry a short heading or 'running head'. This heading is usually the same as the heading of the main chapter or section in which the page falls. Running heads are useful for readers flipping through the document looking for a specific section, and to remind them which section they are currently looking at. The footer zone is an equivalent area at the bottom of the page, but this is less commonly used for 'headings'.

Most publications have either headers or footers but not both, simply because they encroach on the area remaining for the main body of the text. The page number, however, may be included in the header zone, or it may be placed in a footer zone. Header and footer text should be clearly separated spatially from the main text, and it should be typographically distinguished in some way. A smaller type size will prevent any confusion with headings in the body of the text. If a contrasting typeface is in use for chapter headings, this same face might be used for headers and footers. Italics are another possibility.

The position of the header or footer text in relation to the width of the page should be decided in relation to the grid. It can be ranged against either the left or right margin of the page, or the main text column. The advantage of placing running heads against the outer margin of each page is that they are easy to see as the pages of the document are flicked over.

The position of the page numbers should be determined by the grid, but the closer they are to the outer margin of each page, the more easily they will be seen. Whether they are placed at the top or bottom of the pages will depend on what fits in best with the header or footer text and with other aspects of the page layout.

Preliminary pages

The preliminary pages should be designed according to the same principles as the rest of the publication. The grid should either be the same as that used for the main text, or should be closely related to it.

The title page is conventionally a righthand page. The appearance of the title on the title page is usually more emphatic than the chapter headings. Sometimes the design of the title page is simply a repeat of the typographic elements on the cover. Otherwise the positioning of the title should relate to the grid. If chapter headings are placed at a particular level on the page, you may wish to position the title in the same way.

The design of the acknowledgments, preface or foreword, and introduction should echo that of the main text, but you may prefer to use headings that are slightly less emphatic than the main chapter headings. These should relate to headings used for other matter such as the contents list, glossary, index and appendices.

The cover

The design of the cover should relate to the design of the publication as a whole. For example, if an asymmetric layout has been used throughout, then the cover should be asymmetric too.

A simple, uncluttered cover will give maximum impact. You may decide to use typography alone, in which case it should be simple and strong. If you decide to use an image, then it is better to use one reasonably sized image than several small ones. If a publication deals with several different topics, it is usually a mistake to try and illustrate all of them. Readers won't know which image to look at first, and it may take them some time to work out the significance of each. One strong illustration will be much more effective. If necessary the major topics covered can be listed very briefly on the cover. Any photographs or illustrations used must be relevant and technically of a high quality; they must also be well-reproduced.

Page make-up

The grid provides a system for the consistent arrangement of text, tables and illustrations on the page, but it is also important to consider the flow of information from page to page.

Breaking the information into pages causes little problem when a document consists of continuous text only. The main difficulties that are likely to occur are with 'widows' and 'orphans'. The last line of a paragraph is called a widow when it is carried over to the next page. The first line of a paragraph is an orphan if it occurs at the bottom of a page. Both of these situations should be avoided if possible, especially where paragraphs are separated by vertical space. An isolated line — or part of a line in the case of a widow — makes a very untidy end or beginning to a page. The most satisfactory solution is to edit the text slightly so that the problem does not arise. Alternatively, the page can be left short: an orphan can be taken over to the next page, and in the case of the widow, the penultimate line of the paragraph can be taken over to accompany it. You should not try to solve the problem by 'massaging' the vertical spacing on the page, for reasons explained earlier in this chapter.

In text that contains headings and listed points, there is always the risk that a heading will fall at the bottom of page, or that the introduction to a list of points will be separated from the points themselves. The adjustments in vertical spacing that you would need to make to prevent this happening would almost certainly be noticeable, and would undermine your system of spatial cueing. The only satisfactory solution is to leave the page short and take the heading or the introductory sentence over to the next page.

The situation is even more complex when there are tables and illustrations that need to be looked at in relation to particular parts of the text. Each table and illustration should be placed as close as possible to the point where it is referred to. Readers should certainly not be expected to flick back and forth from one page to another to find illustrations or tables if there is any way in which this can be avoided. Occasionally it may be necessary to leave a page short so that the various elements can be brought back in step with one another. Reference to another page may be unavoidable if the same table or illustration is relevant to the text on more than one page. In this case it is usually best to insert the table or illustration when it is first referred to.

To sum up, your main concerns in making up pages should be to ensure that related items (text, tables, illustrations, notes etc.) are as close together as possible, and to preserve consistent spatial cueing. If material has to be taken over to the next page for any reason, it is almost always better to leave the page short rather than spread out the remaining text to fill the page. Similarly, information should not be squeezed onto a page to prevent it from going over onto the next page.

What next?

We suggest that you now go back to your information and examine its structure carefully — particularly if it was written by someone other than yourself. Look at the number and kind of tables and illustrations, and see if there are notes that need integrating page by page with the text. Work out how many levels of heading are needed, how many different kinds of listed points, and so on. Look especially hard for any logical inconsistencies that need correcting. In other words, familiarise yourself thoroughly with the information so that you know what it is that you are trying to represent typographically.

You will then be in a position to devise a tentative scheme. This scheme should provide 'rules' for the treatment of every different kind of information within your document. Draw diagrams and make notes so that you have an accurate record of your scheme.

Then check through your information again to make sure that every part of it fits comfortably within your scheme without any distortion. If there are problems, then you may have to re-think some aspects of your scheme. In extreme cases, however, the only sensible solution may be to treat the problem material as a one-off. For example, if designing all tables to suit the requirements of one particularly difficult example meant that all the other tables suffered visually for the sake of the one, you would be justified in allowing an exception to your rules. Generally speaking, though, you should try to devise a scheme that suits all of your information. Occasionally you will have to look for ingenious ways of re-structuring information, or possibly even modifying its content slightly, but this should never be done at the expense of accuracy or clarity. Information should never be forced into a format that doesn't suit it.

Summary

The logical structure of the text must be made clear to your readers. White space, and variations in type size, style and face, can be used to emphasise, divide and relate information. The same basic principles can be applied to all the various text structures that are likely to occur within a document, from continuous text to complex tables, bibliographies and indexes. It is also important to ensure that related text, tables and illustrations are brought together at the page make-up stage. Consistency in the treatment of similar kinds of information within the document is essential for an easy-to-understand and professional-looking result. Before you begin to 'design' your document, you should devise a set of design 'rules' covering all the different kinds of text structure that occur, rather than making one-off decisions as the need arises.

DESIGNING IN COLOUR

6

The dimensions of colour and colour mixing. How colour is generated on the VDU screen. Primary and secondary methods of producing colour hard copy. Specifying colour. Colour and legibility.
Using colour on projected images and on paper. Using colour to
show the structure of the data — emphasis and colour coding.
Making the best use of colour in text and tables and in diagrams,
charts and graphs.

Introduction

Colour undoubtedly increases the attention-attracting qualities
of a printed document, poster or slide, but its value as part of the
communication process depends on how it is used. Well used, it
can make the structure of the information much clearer and the
display as a whole more attractive. Badly used, it can result in
images that are illegible, confusing and ugly.

Colour is a powerful grouping cue and can be used very effectively to emphasise, divide and relate information. Even if the
colour was not applied with this purpose in mind, people will
still look for similarities between items in the same colour, and for
differences between items in different colours. They will be confused if the colour carries no meaning. Colour must therefore be
used logically and consistently, and with restraint. Colour used
merely as decoration, i.e. without function, has no place in scientific presentation.

The dimensions of colour

Colour is described in terms of three dimensions:

*   *Hue.* The human visual system perceives different wave-
    lengths of light as different colour sensations. Hue is that

property of a colour that depends on its dominant wave-length, i.e. the wavelength most heavily represented in the colour. Hue is described by terms such as red, blue, green, etc..

- *Saturation.* The term 'saturation' relates to the purity of a colour. Highly saturated colours consist of only a narrow band of wavelengths. Unsaturated colours have various quantities of other wavelengths mixed in with them. This is the equivalent of adding white.

- *Lightness.* Colours can be placed on a scale from dark to light. On the computer screen, where light is transmitted rather than reflected, the term usually used is 'brightness'.

Additive and subtractive colour mixing

Colour on a computer-driven VDU is generated by the additive mixing of light in three primary colours: red, green and blue. With additive mixing, the more colours you add the lighter the mixture becomes. Mixtures of two additive primary colours give the additive complementaries: red plus green gives yellow, red plus blue gives magenta (a bluish red), and green plus blue gives cyan (a greenish blue). The three primaries together give white. The fact that red and green mix to give yellow is especially sur-prising to those who are used to mixing coloured pigments rather than coloured light.

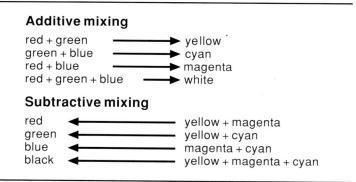

Additive mixing

red + green   ⟶ yellow
green + blue   ⟶ cyan
red + blue   ⟶ magenta
red + green + blue ⟶ white

Subtractive mixing

red   ⟵ yellow + magenta
green   ⟵ yellow + cyan
blue   ⟵ magenta + cyan
black   ⟵ yellow + magenta + cyan

The mixing of pigments is subtractive: the more colours you add, the darker the mixture becomes. This is because pigments absorb some wavelengths of light and reflect others. When two pigments are mixed, the mixture will reflect only those wavelengths that *both* pigments are capable of reflecting; other wavelengths are absorbed. The subtractive primaries are yellow, magenta and cyan. Yellow and magenta mix to give red, because red wave-lengths are the only ones that both pigments are capable of reflecting. Similarly, yellow and cyan mix to give green, and cyan and magenta mix to give blue. Yellow, magenta and cyan together give a brownish black. Subtractive mixing using these colours is the basis of colour printing and colour photography.

Colour on the computer screen

The VDU screen is covered in tiny dots of three different kinds of ***Colour*** phosphor, each dot being capable of emitting either red, green or ***generation*** blue light. The dots are arranged in groups of three, one of each colour. They are so small that the naked eye cannot distinguish them, so light from adjacent dots appears to be mixed. When all of the dots are 'off', the screen appears black. When dots of only one primary colour are 'on', the screen will appear to be that colour. Mixtures of two primaries give the additive complementaries, and when all of the dots are switched on at their full luminance (or brightness), the screen appears white. By varying the proportions of red, green and blue dots that are on, it is possible to generate a wide range of colours. On most VDUs the luminance of each phosphor dot can be varied too, giving palettes of colours ranging from fully saturated primary hues to pale pastels and darker, muddy shades.

The number of colours you can display will depend on the kind of VDU you have and the software you are using. There may be as few as eight colours available, or as many as 16 million! The basic principles of colour generation are the same, no matter how many colours you have.

Because of the way colours are generated on a VDU, they inevita- ***Relative*** bly differ in their luminance, or brightness. The table gives rela- ***luminances*** tive luminance values for the primaries, complementaries and white. Other mixtures will fall somewhere in between. As we shall see, differences in luminance have consequences for legibility, and for the use of colour as a way of giving emphasis.

VDU Colour	Relative luminance %
White	100
Yellow	89
Cyan	70
Green	59
Magenta	41
Red	30
Blue	11

Creating hardcopy in colour

When you create work on a VDU screen you are 'painting with light'. There is no way that any form of hardcopy can truly emulate screen effects. The nearest you can get to adequate reproduction of screen colour is to print directly onto colour film via a dedicated film printer to make slides or overhead projection transparencies. Photographing the screen is only useful for draft quality work.

Coloured images can be generated directly from your computer by a variety of means (primary methods), or you can add colour to black-and-white images later (secondary methods).

Primary methods The direct methods of creating hard copy in colour are as follows:

- On a colour plotter.

- On a colour laserprinter, dye sublimation printer, or wax colour printer. The wax process gives transparent colours of great intensity which are particularly suitable for overhead projection transparencies and the making of slides from printed hardcopy.

- Via a slide printer.

Secondary methods If you don't have access to one of the above printing methods, black laserprinter and photocopier images may be coloured via a secondary colour transfer process:

- By printing onto coloured paper.

- By adding transparent or opaque self-adhesive sheets.

- By bonding coloured carbon particles to the existing black images. For example, in the Omnichrom™ system, coloured sheets of carbon are sandwiched with the existing artwork and the colour is fixed to the black images by heat.

When you are creating the image on your computer screen, it is important to work in the final mode of presentation. In other words, if you are intending your work to be seen in black and white, don't work in colour and vice versa.

Specifying colours

Drawing and illustration programs will typically offer you at least four ways of specifying the colours you use in your computer artwork. The best method to use will depend on what form the output will take, and on which method you find easiest to use.

The most commonly used systems are:

- RGB (Red, Green, Blue)

- HLS (Hue, Lightness, Saturation)

- Pantone
- CMYK (Cyan, Magenta, Yellow, Black)

In the RGB system, a colour is described in terms of the output **RGB**
from the three electron guns responsible for activating the red,
green and blue phosphors. A percentage value is given for each
gun. Thus R100%/G100%/B0% would be a fully saturated yellow. This system is simple to use for primary and complementary
colours, but if you are not used to it you may find it difficult to
imagine what values are needed to create more subtle colours.

The HLS system is more intuitive. Hues are thought of as being **HLS**
arranged in a colour circle and are specified in degrees from 0 to
360. Red is at 0°, yellow at 60°, green at 120°, cyan at 180°, blue at
240° and magenta at 330°. Lightness is specified as a percentage,
as is saturation. A disadvantage of this system, however, is that
lightness and saturation are not independent. A primary green,
for example, would be maximally saturated at a lightness of 50%.
This would be the equivalent of a value of 100% on the 'green'
gun in the RGB system. Lightness can be increased further only
by a contribution from the other two guns. This is the equivalent
of adding white. Saturation is therefore reduced.

The RGB and HLS systems work well if you are copying your
work direct to slide. You may find that the colours on the slides do
not precisely match those on your VDU, but they will be quite
close. If there is a marked difference, your screen may need cali-
brating. The manuals for some programs include a colour chart
and instructions to help you do this. RGB and HLS cannot be used
if your work is to be printed. The colours will have to be converted to one of the colour print systems such as Pantone or
CMYK equivalents (see below), and although your program will
do this for you, the equivalents are not always exact.

The Pantone system relates to a range of coloured inks used in ***Pantone***
printing. It is possible to obtain books and colour swatches which
give printed examples of all the Pantone colours, each of which
has a number. If you need to print only four or fewer different colours, you can simply specify the appropriate Pantone numbers
from your printed colour swatch. It is possible that when you
specify the same Pantone numbers on your VDU the colours may
not exactly match the swatch, but this won't matter. The colour on
screen is simply to give you an indication of what the printed illustration will look like.

Pantone colours are printed as 'spot' colours, i.e. each colour is
printed with a different ink. If you need to print more than four
colours, it will be more economical to use the CMYK system of
'process' colours rather than spot colours. This is because printing presses can print a maximum of only four spot colours at one

time, whereas with process colours it is possible to reproduce an enormous range of colours using only four inks. The process colours are the subtractive primaries — cyan, magenta and yellow — plus black. Black is used because the cyan, magenta and yellow alone do not give a dense black.

Process colours: CMYK Process printing involves the preparation of four separate pieces of artwork for each colour image, known as colour separations. Colour separations are the equivalent of taking black and white photographs of the image through red, green and blue filters. At the same time, the image is broken up into dots using a halftone screen. The separations are used to make four printing plates, each of which is printed with a different process colour.

If you want to use process printing to produce a specific Pantone colour, you will find that Pantone books and swatches give the CMYK values for each colour. Alternatively, your program may convert Pantone colours to CMYK values for you. Process printing can also be used to create high quality reproductions of colour photographs and continuous tone (see Glossary) colour artwork. However, using process colours involves making colour separations. Although page make-up programs can do this automatically, it is best left to the professionals.

Colour and legibility

Contrast There are several factors that affect the legibility of coloured lettering and other small coloured images such as lines and symbols. Perhaps the most important of these is the light/dark contrast between foreground and background. It is not enough to use two colours that are very different in hue. There must also be a strong light/dark or luminance contrast, because the eye and brain rely mainly on luminance differences to locate the edges of foreground images. Hue plays very little part. Cyan text on a yellow background is very difficult to read because the luminances of the colours are very close. On a light background, dark or low-luminance colours will be the most legible, with black giving the best legibility, whereas on a dark background, light or high-luminance colours will work best.

Chromatic aberration Hue does have some effect on legibility. Primary red and blue are not very satisfactory as foreground colours on VDUs, slides and OHPs because of the effects of chromatic aberration. Different wavelengths of light are bent by different amounts as they pass through the eye, so if white is in focus on the retina, then blue will come to a focus in front of it and red behind it. This results in blurred images for the out-of-focus colours. There is also a stereoscopic depth effect whereby pure red and pure blue images appear to be in different planes. The effect can be disturbing when red and blue are used close to one another on a dark background.

Primary blue is particularly unsuitable for use as an image col-   *Avoid primary*
our. Apart from the effects of chromatic aberration, the eye is less   *blue as an*
sensitive to blue than to other colours (which will make the blue   *image colour*
look darker), and the visual acuity (resolving power) of the eye is
lower for blue than for other colours. Again, the effects are particularly marked when blue is used on a dark background.

All of these effects are much more noticeable when the medium is
transmitted light (VDUs) as compared with reflected light
(printed paper).

Using colour on slides and OHPs

Dark lettering on a light background will give better legibility   *Background*
than light lettering on a dark background. This is because small   *colour*
bright images on a dark background appear to spread and blur, as
we explained on page 44. If you have a special reason for using a
dark background, remember to choose a typeface with open
counters, and to check that the letter spacing is adequate.

If you choose a light background, don't use a pure white or the re-
sultant glare may cause discomfort. Light pastel colours work
well with black text, but if you are using colour to code lines or
symbols you will do better to choose a neutral background such
as white or very light grey. Darker greys may not give enough
contrast with the lettering colour or colours.

Bright, highly saturated colours are not a good idea for backgrounds because they cause afterimages. If your audience has to
look at, say, a bright green background for 20 seconds or so and
you then show them a slide with a white background, the white
will look pink. (The colour of the afterimage is always the complementary of the stimulus colour.) Primary blue backgrounds
should be avoided where legibility is critical.

If possible, all of your slides should have backgrounds of about
the same brightness, or your audience will be constantly having
to re-adapt their eyes.

The impact of foreground colours depends very much on the   *Foreground*
choice of background colour. Coloured images on a light ground   *colour*
must be drawn thicker and lettering must be bolder and larger
than the same images on a dark ground.

As we have explained, good contrast between foreground and
background is one of the most important factors for legibility.
Thus dark colours need light backgrounds, and vice versa. If the
foreground and background colours are similar in lightness, optical interference effects may be created. Red lettering on grey of
a similar lightness is particularly difficult to read, as are pairs of
complementary colours such as red and blue-green.

Muddy blues, greens, browns and pinks tend not to work well as foreground colours on slides. Although we are recommending low-saturation colours for slide backgrounds, foreground colours need to be highly saturated if they are to be discriminated from one another. It must also be remembered that colour saturation on slides can be seriously reduced by inadequate power from the projector lamp, and by stray light falling on the screen.

Using colour on paper

The legibility of coloured lettering on white paper will depend largely on the lightness contrast of the pigment with the paper. Black therefore remains the most legible colour on white paper; yellow is the least legible. For good legibility, the contrast between pigment and paper should be at least 70%. Strongly coloured papers should be avoided because they will reduce contrast and hence legibility. Conversely, if you are using white type reversed out of a coloured background, the darker the background the more legible the type will be.

If you are thinking of using colour, it is important to bear in mind the consequences if the original is likely to be copied in black and white. Xerographic copiers vary in their ability to reproduce colours. They may copy strong colours quite successfully, but some machines copy blue well, others copy red well. Very few will reproduce both well.

Colour for emphasis

The amount of emphasis conveyed by a colour depends on its contrast with the background. The greater the contrast, the greater the impact of the colour. The most emphatic colours should therefore be used for the most important information, in the same way that bold type or a larger type size might be used. If you ignore this principle, your audience may be confused by the apparent emphasis of unimportant information.

With a white background, therefore, the darker the colour the more dominant it will seem. Black and other dark colours will give most emphasis, while lighter colours such as yellow will give the least. Although red is usually considered to have impact, lettering or lines in black and in the same size will generally appear stronger. Any coloured texts will need to be larger than the same texts in black. The degree of contrast between one object and another is always more important than differences in colour.

With black backgrounds, it is the lighter colours that dominate. Taking the primary VDU colours and their complementaries, white and yellow are among the most dominant colours, followed by colours such as cyan and green. Red is one of the least dominant colours on a black background, so its usefulness as a means of attracting attention to important items is questionable.

Colour coding

Colour coding is simply a way of grouping words or images by colour. If it is to be successful, the colours in the set must be easy to discriminate from one another.

Saturation is an important factor in colour discrimination. Highly saturated reds, oranges, yellows, greens and blues are easier to discriminate from one another than less saturated colours.

Discrimination is also affected by the lightness or luminance contrast between the image and the background. Coloured lines on a bright white background will appear darker and less saturated than the same lines on a black background. If they appear so dark and desaturated that it is difficult to tell them apart, try making them a little lighter. With black backgrounds, the opposite problem can sometimes occur: light colours may appear washed out and difficult to tell apart, so they may need to be made a little darker. Colour discrimination on both white and black backgrounds will be improved by using colours that differ in lightness as well as in hue, but bear in mind that this may result in apparent differences of emphasis.

Colour discrimination

If it is essential that the audience should be able to discriminate between small areas of colour on slides, it may be wiser to use a black background, but not if this means mixing dark and light backgrounds in the same series of slides.

The size of the coloured areas is important too, because the human eye is not capable of discriminating accurately between small areas of colour. As the area diminishes, so colour effects are lost and only light/dark differences remain. This will be especially true for graph lines or small lettering or symbols on a white background, where colour discrimination will also be impaired by the contrast effect mentioned above. Thus a thin blue line and a thin red line will both appear to be 'dark' and may be very difficult to tell apart. This difficulty can be counteracted to some extent by increasing the line thickness and the stroke thickness of lettering on white backgrounds.

A further difficulty may arise if colour-coded symbols appear on different backgrounds in the same display. The apparent colour of the symbols will be shifted towards the complementary colour of the background. For example, the same white may appear yellowish on a blue background, greenish-blue on a red background, and pinkish on a green background. These effects will be most marked with symbols in relatively light, unsaturated colours.

How many Don't use more than seven colours in a colour coding scheme, or
colours? users will find it difficult to discriminate between them if the
whole set is not available for comparison. Even with smaller sets
of colours, they may forget the significance of a particular colour.

For most purposes, four is a realistic number of colours to use.
These colours should be as different as possible in hue. Blue and
green, for example, might easily be confused because they are
relatively close in hue. The risk of confusion could be reduced by
choosing a blue towards the violet end of the spectrum, and a yellowish green. A lightness difference would make discrimination
easier still.

Colour vision Whenever possible, colour coding should be used as a way of re-
problems inforcing a grouping that has already been made clear in some
other way. Problems of colour discrimination and memory make
it too risky to rely on colour alone. There are also the colour blind
to consider. In the UK about 8% of men and 0.4% of women have
some form of colour vision defect, the most common being a difficulty in discriminating between reds and greens. Some people
have problems in discriminating muddy blues and greens. With
graphics these problems can be partially overcome by using colours that differ in lightness as well as in hue, or by using mechanical tones such as stippling or cross-hatching to distinguish between different areas.

Colour coding is of limited use in text or tables, but it can be invaluable as a way of distinguishing between lines or areas in
charts, graphs and diagrams.

Colour in text and tables

Colour is usually unnecessary in printed text and tables. Spatial
and typographic cueing are more than adequate to make the
structure of the information clear, and there is no point in using
colour for the sake of it. In some situations, though, colour can be
used both meaningfully and as a way of giving added visual interest, especially on slides.

Text Sometimes it can be appropriate to use a second colour for headings. Coloured headings are often used to create visual interest
and aesthetic appeal in magazines and prestige publications. In
public information leaflets, colour may be used to make the information seem more accessible and palatable. Coloured headings
can be helpful on slides too. Remember that on a white background the colour will be less emphatic than the black text, so you
will need to compensate for this by using a larger size of lettering
for the coloured headings. Alternatively, you might consider su-
perimposing a heading on a panel of background colour. It is important to remember that the lettering and background colours

must differ considerably in lightness or luminance if the wording is to be legible.

On slides it may very occasionally be appropriate to use colour to emphasise particular words in the text, in the same way that italics might be used in print. Restraint is the keyword here. Don't use more than one colour, and don't emphasise more than two or three words per slide. If too many things are emphasised, your audience won't know where to look first and the impact will be lost. The effect is perfectly described in these lines from Gilbert and Sullivan's 'The Gondoliers':

'When everyone is somebodee
Then no one's anybody'

Think very carefully before highlighting a whole paragraph in a different colour. You should do this only if the paragraph requires a different level of emphasis (such as an introductory paragraph, or a paragraph summarising important points), and not just because it happens to deal with a different topic. If your main text is in black on a white ground, you may find that the coloured paragraph looks *less* important because of its reduced contrast. You may need to compensate for this by using bold lettering, but bold lettering in black would be even more effective as a way of emphasising the paragraph.

Although colour is unnecessary in printed tables, it can occasion- **Tables**
ally be useful as a way of making a particular point on a slide. Alternatively, it can be used to emphasise the structure of the table. Column and row headings, for example, might be distinguished from the data in the body of the table.

If you are thinking of using colour, remember the following:

- If you want to use colour to draw attention to a particular cell of a table, or a particular row, the remainder of the table must be in one colour only or the impact will be lost.

- Don't use different colours for different columns just because they contain different kinds of information. This will draw the eye down the table instead of across.

- Resist the temptation to use two colours on alternate lines of a table as a way of guiding the eye across. Striped tables have been tested against single-colour versions, and the stripes were found to be distracting and of no help. If you feel that it will be difficult for your audience to read across a table, your layout is at fault.

- Don't use more than two colours in any table.

Colour in diagrams, graphs and charts

If colour has no direct purpose of its own in your work, don't use it. The only exception to this is that if all your slides in a presentation are colour slides, then diagrams in black and white may look out of place. Even in these cases it is still better to create data in colour monochrome, i.e. use just one colour as a background and a second colour for the images.

Bar graphs Colour can sometimes be a useful way of coding bars or bar segments in bar graphs, though if the colours are not fairly close together in lightness or luminance, differences in importance may be implied. With similar lightnesses, however, the colour coding may be confusing for those with colour vision defects. The answer is not to rely on colour coding alone, but to use it in addition to other cues. Ideally the bars should also be clearly labelled.

Colour can also be used as a way of drawing attention to data points that exceed a particular value. The bars would then need to be all the same colour, with a second colour where any bar exceeds a given value.

Line graphs Colour is especially useful with multi-line graphs. Unless lines are adequately coded and crossing points clearly indicated, monochrome multi-line graphs can be ambiguous. With coloured lines, the axes, scale calibrations and all labels should ideally be in some neutral colour such as black on a white background (or white on a black background). Sometimes, though, it can be difficult to directly label the lines because of lack of space. It may then be helpful to colour the labels to match the lines. As a guide, coloured lines on a white ground should be at least three times thicker than they would need to be if they were in black.

Summary

Use colour logically and with restraint. Specify colours by the method best suited to your output medium. Coloured lettering and backgrounds affect legibility. You must ensure that there is a strong light/dark contrast between foreground and background. In general, light backgrounds with dark type give better legibility than dark backgrounds with light type. Slides in the same series should all have backgrounds of similar brightness. Colour can be used for emphasis and for coding. Colours that have the greatest light/dark contrast with the background will have the strongest impact. Colour coding is often helpful in multi-line graphs and other kinds of diagram. Remember that viewers will look for relationships between items in the same colour.

DIAGRAMS AND GENERAL DRAWING TIPS

7

Computer generated artwork differs greatly from the pen and paper kind. Computers use three main ways to deal with images: bitmapping, vector mapping and pathway mapping. All objects can be constructed from three basic forms. How to use these to create diagrams. Tips for drawing tubes, spirals, genomes, equations and DNA structures. Storing images and styles created by a drawing/illustration/wordprocessing program in either the 'Scrapbook' or as a 'Stationery' document for repeated use.

New ways of thinking

Artwork creation on a computer requires a totally different way of thinking from that which would be used for work using pen, ink and paper. There are two major differences. Firstly, computer drawings start from manipulating a few very elementary geometric figures: the line (or pathway), the square, the circle and the triangle. All other shapes are made by manipulating these primary elements. The second difference is that the finished drawing simply metamorphoses out of the original and subsequent drafts. A very useful part of computer artwork is that you can store each stage of a drawing as it progresses so that you can get back to any one of them if need be.

The creative power offered by computers to artists is virtually unlimited. We are free, at last, from the constraints imposed by materials. There is nothing to stand between you and the creation of your ideas. There are, of course, some limiting factors that may be mildly annoying, such as the size of the screen or memory limitations of the computer. But you soon learn to accept these in preference to the pen that clogs up, the paper that smudges, and, as we pointed out in the introduction to this book, the dog that puts its muddy paws on the drawing or eats it.

How computers draw images

'Paint' programs

There are basically three ways that computers draw images. First, bitmapping. At the least sophisticated end, this is how most entry level 'paint' programs work. In effect a drawing consists of black dots (pixels) on the screen, which are placed there in a chequerboard fashion. Where these appear to touch, a shape is created. These programs can be fun but their images are at a low resolution of approximately 75 dots per inch.

Bitmapping: dots are placed chequerboard fashion via an invisible grid

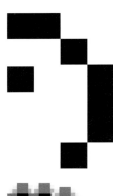

Sophisticated bitmapping: the dots are 'anti-aliased' to produce an effect of smoothness

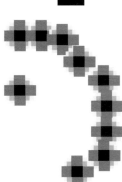

There are also sophisticated bitmap paint programs which can produce very fine images by a system of dithering the dots so that smooth lines and gradations of tone or colour are created. Most of these programs are very expensive and use a lot of memory . They are not normally needed for life-science illustrations such as you see in many journals. Paint programs normally store work as bitmap files. Drawings done in a paint program can be edited only in a paint program. All paint images are homogeneous, in the sense that once an image is committed to the electronic paper it cannot be remodelled or reconstituted into its different parts.

'Draw' programs

Second are the 'draw' images which are produced by vector mapping. The drawing principle in vector mapping is based on establishing dots at a location within the electronic space, defined by a system of co-ordinates. This allows the dots to overlap, and much smoother drawings are possible.

Vector mapping: dots are sent to coordinates

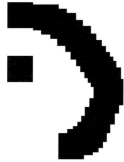

Everything in the draw environment is an object, even space. These objects are separate entities, thus every unit of the drawing can be disconnected from other units and edited at any time. In one sense the images cannot be destroyed by having other images put on top of them, so they can be combined or separated again as you wish. This is something quite impossible in the old world of pen and paper. These programs produce 'publisher acceptable' quality images when the output devices deliver 300dpi or more.

Images created in draw programs are generally stored as PICT or
TIFF files. (These are acronyms for the computer languages used
for writing the image to disc.) But there is a problem here. There
are a number of types of PICT and they are *not* always compatible
with each other. It is therefore important when using a draw program to save a copy of the drawing in its native format. This
means: in the normal mode of the program.

Sometimes you may be offered the choice of saving for export in
PICT , TIFF or some other format. Any 'save' procedure in a non-
native format may lose you essential data from the original. However saving in a non-native format is often needed when export-
ing to other programs.

Every time you save an image in another format, make sure you
give it a new name, otherwise you can over-write (destroy) the
original. Thus, if you make a drawing in MacDraw™ and call it
'Test tube', and then you want to export a copy to another program such as PageMaker™, which may only accept TIFF images,
you would save the export version as 'Test tube TIFF'.

Thirdly there are the 'illustration' programs. These produce the highest level of
drawing using pathway mapping. This is
quite a different system again. Illustration
programs such as FreeHand™ and Illus-
trator™ provide the most sophisticated
drawing possible. They are capable of producing the finest and smoothest of lines.
In simple terms, objects are drawn as pathways. These pathways have no dimensions, they are purely abstract.

When a pathway has been established, a
subsequent series of commands then tells
the pathway what to do with itself. This
might be to draw as black, as white, as a
tone, as a colour and be of a certain thickness (width). Likewise with the filling of
enclosed shapes. They may or may not
have an outline, they can be filled with
nothing, white, black, tone, colour, gradu-
ations of tone and colour, or with patterns.

Further instructions will tell the pathway
to connect to other pathways. These instructions are embedded in a sophisticated computer language such as
PostScript™. Because of its greater complexity, pathway mapping uses more
memory than vector mapping. However,

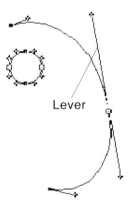

**'Illustration'
programs**

A pathway is
established.
This is purely
abstract.
The levers control
the curves

Lever

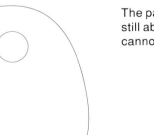

The pathways are
still abstract ,so
cannot be printed

The pathways are given a thickness and a tone value. Now they have substance and can be printed

the quality of the image held in the computer is 'perfect' and is only limited by the output device, i.e. the printing engine or slide/transparency printer.

Unfortunately the computer screen only provides a 'representation' of the image at 75dpi. You have to have a printer's proof to see how good it is. Images created by illustration programs are normally stored as encapsulated PostScript files (EPS). However they can also be exported as PICT or TIFF files and so used in other 'draw' programs.

EPS files retain all the information relating to the image and so are infinitely editable. If the original EPS drawing is exported or filed in PICT or TIFF format, some of the information in the original drawing may be lost; typically this applies to complex shading.

Basic geometry of all objects

When you draw with a computer instead of a pen, you have to think differently and often a lot more clearly. For instance, next time you look at any apparently complicated drawing or diagram, ask yourself: 'What are the basic geometric units involved?' It will be unusual if there are more than three: a triangle, a rectangle and a circle. The cone is only a three-dimensional representation of a triangle. The cylinder is the same of a rectangle and the sphere is the same of a circle.

All that exists in this world is constructed of these three basic shapes

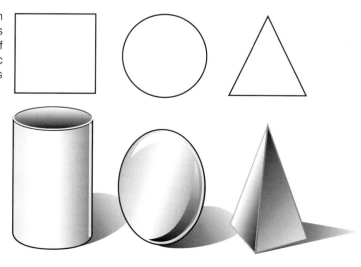

The pictures on the previous page were produced in the illustration program FreeHand™. The shading is computer controlled. To get the best out of these programs, we admit that it helps to understand the basics of drawing, such as perspective and the use of shading and shadow. Apart from extra drawing control, the advantage of using illustration programs is that they allow you to produce the best quality output that your printer is capable of. But these programs tend to be expensive and are only worth it if you are going to do a lot of drawings and you want the quality.

Elementary diagrams

The illustrations on this page show how effective diagrams can be made quickly by manipulating the same basic components in

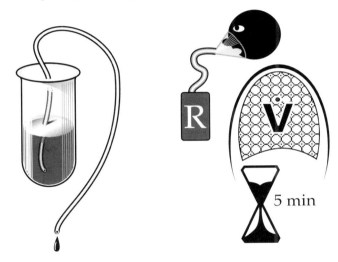

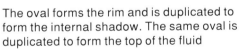

The oval forms the rim and is duplicated to form the internal shadow. The same oval is duplicated to form the top of the fluid

This shape, derived from the triangle, forms the shadow by having no outline and a graduated fill

This is the fluid, filled with tone made from duplicating the test tube and then cutting it in half

These bars are drawn from a single line duplicated, one set being drawn in white and one in grey

This is the half outline

different ways. The test tube is made from just five elements. To emphasise the new way of thinking, look at how the test tube itself is constructed from only one of its halves. The half is cloned (a copy is placed exactly over the original), and this is then reflected (flipped) on its vertical axis and the two halves joined. It is the work of seconds. Tubing is a different story, as explained below.

The diagram of a patient undergoing a ventilation test is as self-explanatory as possible. Only a little extra text would be needed to complete the story. The drawing has been made using the basic units described. For example, the head, the nose, the mouth and the eye were all drawn from the *same* circle by duplicating, resizing and reshaping it.

Tubing

To draw a pair of lines exactly parallel with pen and ink used to be a daunting task, even for experts. Computer graphics has made this very easy. The illustration programs provide the most control but a similar technique can also be applied to all the draw programs. We used FreeHand™ to do these illustrations.

The pathway

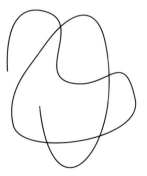

- Draw a pathway representing the shape you want.

- Cut the pathway at the points indicated by the thin lines and deal with these crossing points first.

- Decide how thick you want the tube to be. (Selecting sizes in multiples of two points helps.) In this case we chose 8 points. Paint the pathway with black.

- Clone this line, putting an identical copy over it, reduce the size to 6 points, then paint the new line grey.

- Clone again, reduce the thickness to 2 points and paint in white.

Deciding where to cut the pathway

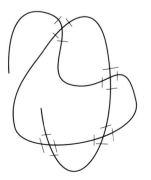

- From each crossing set, decide which of these is to appear below. Select the topmost pathway in this set, the white one, and send it to the back. Do the same with the grey pathway, then the black one. All this set will now appear below the set which crosses it above.

- When this operation has been completed for all the cross sets, you can then proceed to paint and clone the remaining pathways with the same thicknesses and tones as you used for the crossing portions.

Some minor adjustments may be needed to make sure the pathways all remain in contact at their ends, particularly if the cuts are made on a curve.

Perfecting the alignment of pathways needs to be competed *before* cloning takes place. FreeHand™ and Illustrator™ make this easy by allowing you to look at the drawing in 'wire frame mode'. This feature shows the illustration as pathways only and temporarily removes the thicknesses, tones, colours etc..

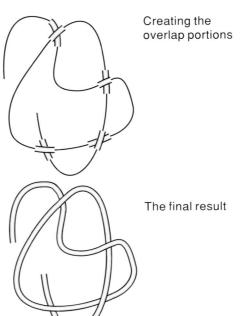

Creating the overlap portions

The final result

Spirals

Spirals can be made from only two units. In this case we have used MacDraft™ since it has the facility for drawing ellipses and elliptical arcs.

The first unit is an elliptical arc, with its cut ends in vertical alignment. This is duplicated and flipped on its vertical axis so that a mirror image is made.

The lower end of one of the arcs is stretched apart and you can then see that by repeating this procedure several times and placing the appropriate arc in contact with its opposite companion, a spiral of any length can be made.

The second unit in the drawing is the small white arcs which are shown on the black ground. These are used to cover over those parts of each arc as it passes under the one above. This little trick should always be used when apparently crossing lines are in fact separated in space. It gives an illusion of perspective and depth.

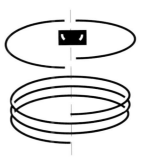

Genomes

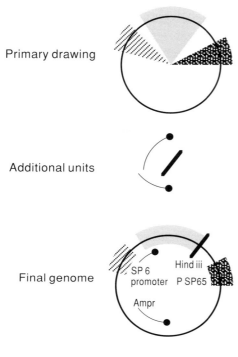

Primary drawing

Additional units

Final genome

Genomes illustrate the genetic endowment of chromosomes. The arc-control tools of MacDraft™ are ideal for creating genomes. You can draw arcs from the centre of any circle and then expand or contract them by pulling the outer corners of the arc.

- First a circle is drawn and, from its centre, arcs are drawn beyond the edge of the circle.

- These arcs are filled with a tone and their outlines are then removed, thus creating wedge shapes.

- A smaller circle filled with white (and finally with no outline) is then placed over the centre, and other items are added and arranged as needed.

Most drawing and illustrating programs have a 'snap to grid' or 'snap to point' feature which allows you to place images *exactly* over any point, making accurate work easy.

Equations

MathType™ is a highly recommended, stand-alone maths program designed to deal with equations, providing full editing control of matrices and automatically expanding brackets. A version of it is incorporated in Microsoft Word™.

An equation built up from a matrix in MathType™

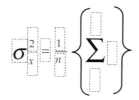

The matrix system is shown on the left. Each dotted outline represents an independent wordprocessing area (the dots are non-printing). However, you can make equations very adequately with any drawing or illustration program. They can then be saved in the Scrapbook for future use in any other document.

This equation was made in MacDraft™, a drawing program

$$\sigma\frac{2}{x} = \frac{1}{n}\left\{\sum_{i=1}^{n} X^2 - n\overline{X}^2\right\}$$

DNA structures

DNA structures often seem difficult to draw, but not if you follow the procedures below. We used FreeHand™.

Use a square with a diagonal as a foundation. Draw a circle centred on a corner of the square, with the circumference passing through the centre of the square. Cut the circle where it intersects the top side of the square and where it intersects the diagonal. Discard all the circle except the 1/8 segment shown in the drawing. This is all you need to build a DNA ribbon, just one element!

Clone and vertically reflect this element and stretch it to the corners of the square. Straighten the curve at the centre so that the transition from the upper curve to the lower one is smooth. Clone the result and move downwards. Shade the resulting form: one copy darker, one copy lighter. Reflect one of these copies on its vertical axis. Then, by duplication, you can create a DNA structure as long as you need and with varying ribbon dispositions.

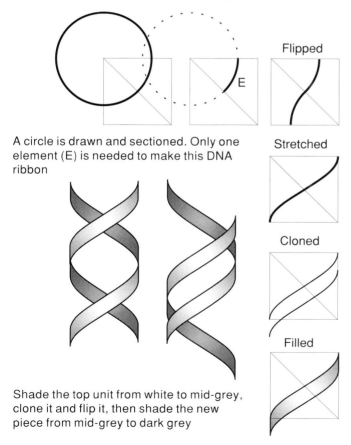

A circle is drawn and sectioned. Only one element (E) is needed to make this DNA ribbon

Flipped

Stretched

Cloned

Filled

Shade the top unit from white to mid-grey, clone it and flip it, then shade the new piece from mid-grey to dark grey

Hierarchical lines

Your eyes automatically assume that a line proceeds in a continuous manner. This assumption can often be wrong. Comparing these two graphs illustrates what we mean.

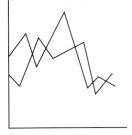

A hierarchy needs to be established so that confusion is avoided. We advocate that in graphs the normal should be emphasised. In other diagrams the main structures should be emphasised.

It is vital in all diagram drawing to decide how objects will be delineated and what scale of importance should be assigned to each.

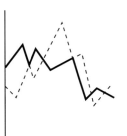

In the test tube diagram (page 97) we chose a thicker line for the test tube itself and the tubing. In the respiration diagram, the time logo was emphasised because this suited the text for which this diagram was made.

Scanners and diagrams

Scanners are essential for the production of the more sophisticated kind of diagram. For example, photographs may be used as a basis for diagrams, sketches and roughs which capture the essential data. They can be used in the background of many drawing and illustration programs so that you can trace over them. Machine traces such as echocardiograms can also be used as a basis for a drawing. Once an image is scanned it can be saved in many of the standard formats such as PAINT, PICT, TIFF or EPS, and so become available to any other program.

Scanners are also useful for capturing text for subsequent optical character recognition (translating typescripts directly to word-processing), or for typographic designs and logos that you may want to use. Scanners are an essential part of the electronic retouching of photographs, using programs like PhotoShop™.

In a sense, scanners are electronic photocopiers and all the same copyright infringement rules apply. Be careful about what you use to base your diagrams on in case you infringe the law. If in doubt, ask, or assume that all work, except your own and that in the public domain, is protected by someone's copyright. (See Chapter 14.)

Area measurement

MacDraft™ possesses a unique feature normally found only in very expensive mathematical programs: the ability to trace complex outlines and calculate the area they enclose. This feature might be very usefully applied to compare cell sizes, the total area relative to the area of the nucleus (shown below), or the changes in area of a particular cell during its lifetime.

The technique used here was to scan a photograph of a cell and import it as a PICT(2) image into MacDraft™, increasing the size to 120% for easier tracing. The program then automatically calculated the area traced. If memory runs low during this process, the outline is traced in sections. The area shown here is correct for the image (on paper) when its Y-axis measures 93.21mm. The actual area at cell level would require further calculation.

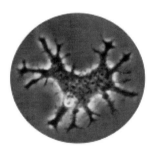

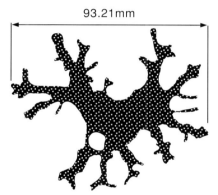

93.21mm

Cell area 2244.58mm²
Nucleus area 62.96mm²

The Scrapbook— a repeatable image store

The Macintosh and Power PC systems incorporate a Scrapbook for keeping any images or text that you may want to use again at a later date. (This is not yet possible with the IBM MS-DOS system or its clones.)

Complex drawings such as family trees are ideal for storage and retrieval. Still more difficult things like twisted DNA molecules can be drawn once, then stored for ever. So can complex formulae. Images kept in the Scrapbook can be copied to new work and modified without destroying the original.

The time saved by using the Scrapbook effectively can be enormous. The Scrapbook normally stores images as bitmaps, PICT or TIFF files. Apart from making your own repeatable images, there is a considerable supply of clip-art or copyright-free images on disc for you to use.

Tip System 7 Scrapbook images are automatically converted to a PICT format. These images often implant into other documents better from the Scrapbook than via other 'export' methods.

Style sheets, stationery or templates

These Scrapbook images are basic units for creating family trees

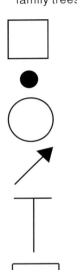

The format of any document can be stored quite apart from its contents. The format is just as much an electronic image as the objects within it.

Saving the format of the first graph you draw will ensure that all the subsequent ones keep the same characteristics (line weights, lettering sizes, types and styles of plotted points). Saving the format of the first poster session you create makes all future work consistent and very much faster. A newsletter is an obvious candidate for a template. It is the best way of retaining a corporate identity.

The manual will tell you how to create stationery and templates. You may be offered an option to save as a template when you save something for the first time. Alternatively, if you go to the File menu and select 'Save as...', you may find the word 'Template' or 'Stationery' there. Clicking on it will save the document, but when it is selected in the future it will show up as 'Untitled'. You are thus forced to save it under a new name. This keeps the original intact for future use.

Why do the same work twice? Examples of templates are: letter headings, forms or form letters, grant applications (if you want to maintain a house style), texts for submission to journals (if you wish to obey their rules consistently), and chapter formats for the book you are writing.

Summary

The creation of successful diagrams depends on choosing the right software for the job. Bitmap, vector map or pathway imaging? Which will work best for you? Your own observation and analysis of the structure of objects can be vital in executing work efficiently. This also means using the particular advantages available only in electronic media such as cloning, enlargement of detail (up to 8 times), snap-to-grid or snap-to-point, saving copies into a Scrapbook, saving styles, reflecting and duplicating. None of these is easily available in the world of pen and ink.

GRAPHS AND CHARTS   8

Understanding how spreadsheet data affect the graph picture. Manipulating graphs beyond the capabilities of the graph program by using 'draw' programs in parallel. Different kinds of graphs and their function. Charts and chemical formulae. Poor graphics and publication refusal. Good graphics and why? Checklist of procedures.

Introduction

Numeric data are usually much better appreciated via pictures. There are many graphing programs that do this. Most of them work on the same principle. The data are entered on a spreadsheet. The first column is normally reserved for the independent variable (category or X axis) and all the other columns are reserved for dependent variables (Y axis). Where this applies in the examples that follow, we have shown a representation of the spreadsheet. By varying the way the data are entered, you will be able to control the way the program draws the graph. How to do a vertical scatter graph is not usually explained in any manuals. Most graph programs offer a considerable choice of graph types as well as a variety of statistical manipulations. You will need to make sure that these satisfy your needs before purchase.

In the best graphing packages the data are 'hot-linked' to the chart drawing so that changes in data automatically cause changes in the drawing. This feature saves a lot of time in those situations where similar data are being often updated. The data can be unlinked if necessary. At an early stage it is important to decide on the presentation format (slide, OHP, poster etc), stretching the graph area as needed before going too far. If the stretching is done later it may lead to distortions of symbols, especially if the graph is imported to a drawing program.

Column and bar graphs

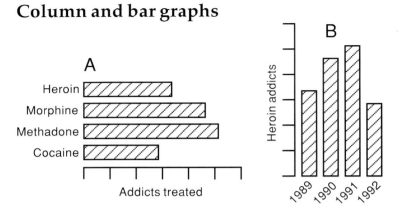

Bar graphs (A) usually compare different variables at the same time or as applied to the same group. Column graphs (B) usually compare the same variable at different times or between different groups. The data are usually discrete or discontinuous.

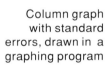

Column graph with standard errors, drawn in a graphing program

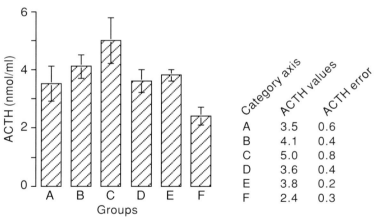

Category axis	ACTH values	ACTH error
A	3.5	0.6
B	4.1	0.4
C	5.0	0.8
D	3.6	0.4
E	3.8	0.2
F	2.4	0.3

Column graphs illustrate discontinuous (discrete) data so the baseline should not be drawn in

Most of the better graph programs will allow you to customise such things as the thickness of the column borders, the fill characteristics of boxes, whether or not the error bars have cross-pieces at either end, plus many other variants. However, there are often occasions when you want more control than is offered in a graphing program, in which case importation into a drawing program is the answer. In the next example we show how the same chart can be transferred to a 'draw' program for modification.

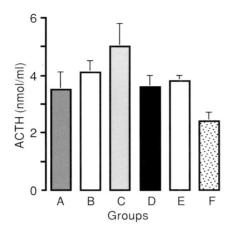

The same graph, transferred to ClarisWorks™ and modified

Note the way standard error bars interfere with the column fills in the graph above. To solve this problem, we have imported the illustration into a 'draw' program where we have complete control over all the elements of the drawing.

In the example below, the boxes we have drawn in around the numbers are simply to emphasise the fact that MVR and AVR are each in two groups of three values. When grouped in this manner, the program will draw the appropriate columns touching each other.

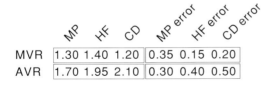

	MP	HF	CD	MP error	HF error	CD error
MVR	1.30	1.40	1.20	0.35	0.15	0.20
AVR	1.70	1.95	2.10	0.30	0.40	0.50

A grouped column graph

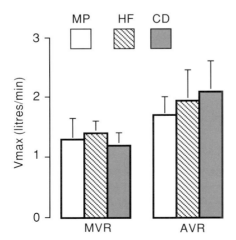

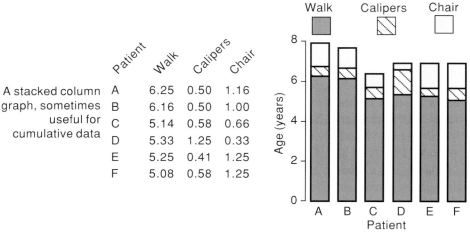

Patient	Walk	Calipers	Chair
A	6.25	0.50	1.16
B	6.16	0.50	1.00
C	5.14	0.58	0.66
D	5.33	1.25	0.33
E	5.25	0.41	1.25
F	5.08	0.58	1.25

A stacked column graph, sometimes useful for cumulative data

Error bars

Some journals may insist on error bars, but the current statistical fashion is to use the mean or deviation and to avoid the often meaningless clutter of standard errors. Most graphing programs such as DeltaGraph™ and CricketGraph™ produce error bars on request. Many spreadsheet programs which may also provide chart options do not allow for automatic error bars; however, there is a trick for producing these, providing you can import the graph into a drawing package later. ClarisWorks™, for example, allows you to do this. We give an outline of the procedure.

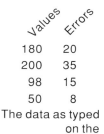

Values	Errors
180	20
200	35
98	15
50	8

The data as typed on the spreadsheet

The data are entered in spreadsheet mode and a stacked bar is selected. In chart options, 'series in columns' is chosen. A stacked column is formed with the top section representing the errors. The graph is transferred to the 'draw' mode where all its parts can be separated by 'ungrouping'. Now the error bars are drawn and placed exactly over the top section of each column. The top sections are then removed, leaving the bars behind.

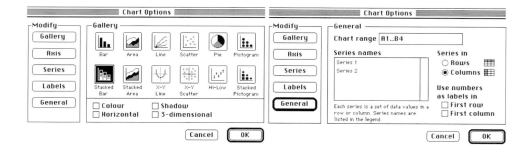

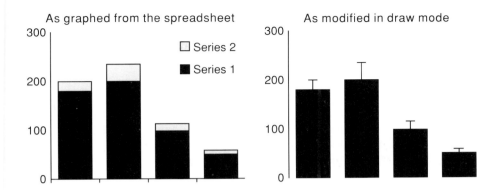

As graphed from the spreadsheet

As modified in draw mode

Enhancements?

Some graphs can be given a three-dimensional look. In column and bar graphs this can give a false impression of the data or obscure it. 3D adds nothing but distraction to a pie graph. Also to be avoided is the jazzy 'Leaning Tower of Pisa' effect caused by diagonal shadings at different angles.

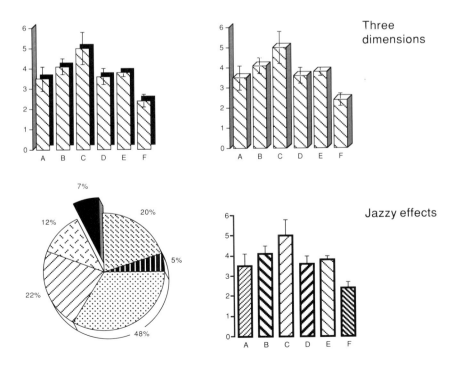

Three dimensions

Jazzy effects

Other forms of column and bar graphs

Histograms compare continuous data in column graph form but at uneven frequencies. It is important to realise that it is the *area* of the rectangles that is measured. Thus the 0-15 age group and the 25-40 age group will contain one third more persons than is indicated by directly measuring off the vertical scale. Histograms are open to misinterpretation if this is not realised. A way around this is to insert the actual number involved at the top of each column

Histogram

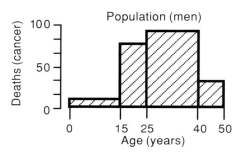

Sliding bar charts are useful for comparing events within the same group and for showing how these compare in turn with similar groups.

Sliding bar graph

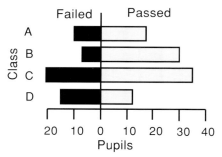

Line graphs

Line graphs illustrate continuous changes of the dependent variable (always plotted on the Y axis) in relation to the independent variable (always plotted on the X axis).

If line graphs have a sufficient number of data points, the line joining them may be curved if the rise and fall is of a continuous nature, such as with temperature. It can be misleading to use a curved line with a small number of data points because there can be no certainty about what happens between widely spaced points.

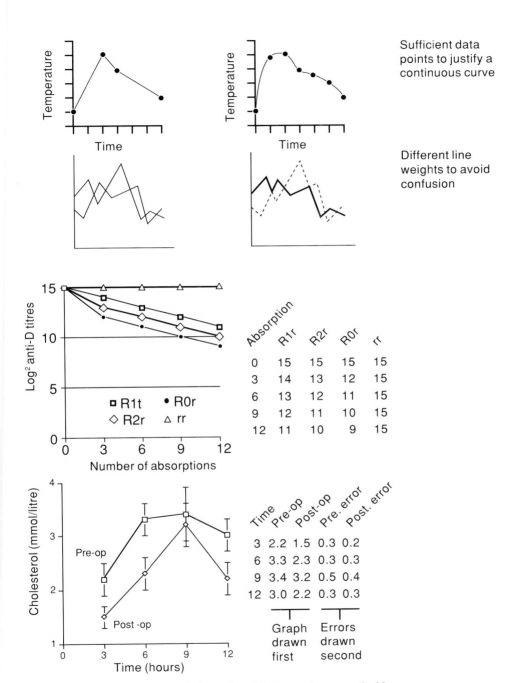

Sufficient data
points to justify a
continuous curve

Different line
weights to avoid
confusion

Absorption	R1r	R2r	R0r	rr
0	15	15	15	15
3	14	13	12	15
6	13	12	11	15
9	12	11	10	15
12	11	10	9	15

Time	Pre-op	Post-op	Pre. error	Post. error
3	2.2	1.5	0.3	0.2
6	3.3	2.3	0.3	0.3
9	3.4	3.2	0.5	0.4
12	3.0	2.2	0.3	0.3

Graph
drawn
first

Errors
drawn
second

If decimal fractions are used, they should always be preceded by
a zero to the left of the decimal point. Overlapping error bars can
be removed or displaced laterally via a drawing program.

Scatter graphs

Scatter graphs normally compare two independent variables, but there may sometimes be a reason to include a third variable on the Z axis.

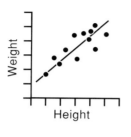 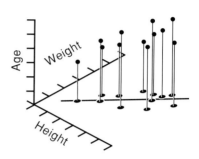

In the following example, a line graph style was selected in the program, not a scatter graph style. The program has automatically set the distance between 'before' and 'after' values.

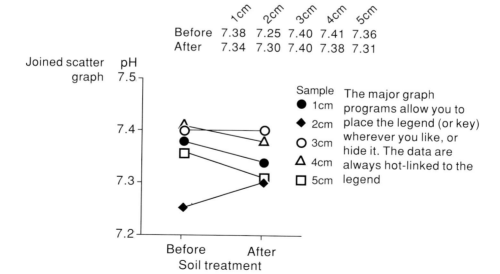

	1cm	2cm	3cm	4cm	5cm
Before	7.38	7.25	7.40	7.41	7.36
After	7.34	7.30	7.40	7.38	7.31

Joined scatter graph

The major graph programs allow you to place the legend (or key) wherever you like, or hide it. The data are always hot-linked to the legend

Vertical scatter and displaced scatter graphs are easy to draw if you use a numeric code in the category (X) axis. The pre-op series in the example below uses the code 1.0, therefore all the dots representing the value (Y) axis will be placed one above the other. The program will allow you to give the dots an outline of white so that overlapping dots are more easily distinguished.

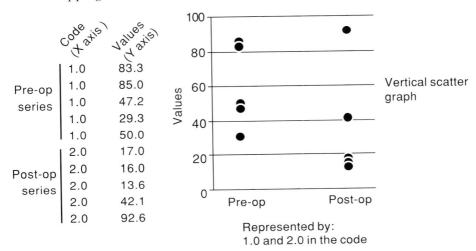

Code (X axis)	Values (Y axis)
Pre-op series	
1.0	83.3
1.0	85.0
1.0	47.2
1.0	29.3
1.0	50.0
Post-op series	
2.0	17.0
2.0	16.0
2.0	13.6
2.0	42.1
2.0	92.6

Vertical scatter graph

Represented by:
1.0 and 2.0 in the code

Our next example shows how to place two or three dots on the same parallel by choosing an X-axis numeral with numbers each side of it. The pre-op series uses a 0.05 difference centred on 2, see (a). The post-op series uses a difference of 0.10 centred on 3, see (b).

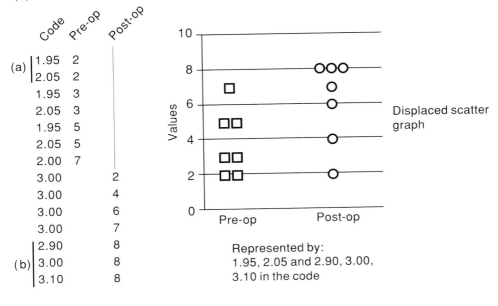

Code	Pre-op	Post-op
(a)		
1.95	2	
2.05	2	
1.95	3	
2.05	3	
1.95	5	
2.05	5	
2.00	7	
3.00		2
3.00		4
3.00		6
3.00		7
(b)		
2.90		8
3.00		8
3.10		8

Displaced scatter graph

Represented by:
1.95, 2.05 and 2.90, 3.00,
3.10 in the code

In the example below we show how two separate plots can be placed within the same graph frame. The program controls the actual placement; all you have to do is make sure that the correct columns of data are selected for each of the sets.

Overlay scatter graph

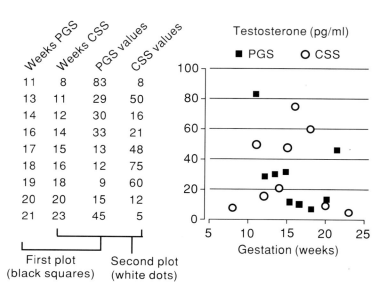

Weeks PGS	Weeks CSS	PGS values	CSS values
11	8	83	8
13	11	29	50
14	12	30	16
16	14	33	21
17	15	13	48
18	16	12	75
19	18	9	60
20	20	15	12
21	23	45	5

First plot (black squares)   Second plot (white dots)

Testosterone (pg/ml)
■ PGS   O CSS

Gestation (weeks)

Pie graphs

Pie graphs are best for illustrating proportions within the whole. No more than eight slices are advised, with the thinnest representing not less than five percent. Most graph programs will allow you to displace slices if you wish to emphasise them and will convert quantities to percentages automatically.

Spreadsheet data

A	50
B	35
C	5
D	10
E	29
F	15
G	2
H	30

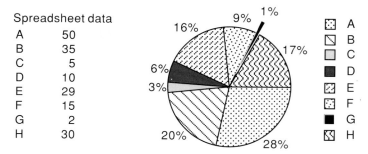

We have deliberately shown one value at 1%. The only way to make this slice show up is to fill it with black and displace it

Polar graphs

Polar graphs portray cyclical data. There may be a difficulty in labelling the concentric axis, but by using markedly different type styles confusion can be avoided.

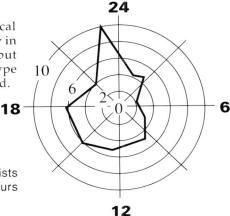

Accidents to cyclists
over 24 hours

Behaviour graphs

Rene Thom's catastrophe theory has been used here to illustrate that small changes in calcium metabolism, seen on the control plane (grid), can cause catastrophic results in the behaviour of bone. Patient (A) remains stable while patient (B) is heading for osteoporosis.

(Data from Prof I Macintyre, RPMS)

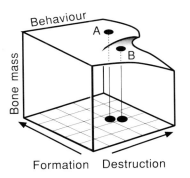

Dendrographs

These graphs compare degrees of similarity between items.

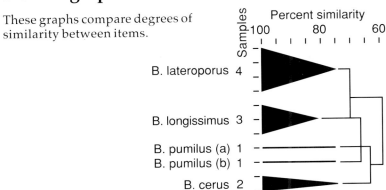

Genealogy charts

Generations should be clearly indicated with roman numerals. Use the symbols shown below. Keep the sizes consistent when making a series of charts in the same publication. Each individual should be identified with arabic numerals placed in a consistent position. The propositus or ego, if known, should always be indicated by an arrow.

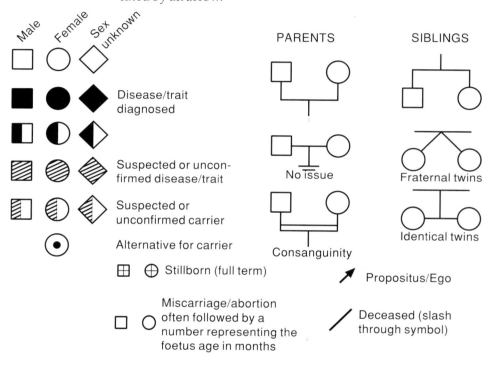

Male Female Sex unknown

PARENTS   SIBLINGS

Disease/trait diagnosed

Suspected or unconfirmed disease/trait   No issue   Fraternal twins

Suspected or unconfirmed carrier

Alternative for carrier   Consanguinity   Identical twins

Stillborn (full term)   Propositus/Ego

Miscarriage/abortion often followed by a number representing the foetus age in months   Deceased (slash through symbol)

Chemical formulae

Always check the house style of the journal you are submitting to and look at their previously published material.

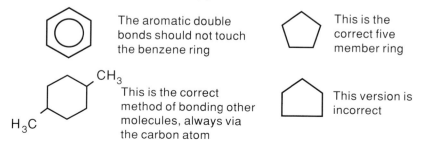

The aromatic double bonds should not touch the benzene ring   This is the correct five member ring

CH₃

This is the correct method of bonding other molecules, always via the carbon atom   This version is incorrect

H₃C

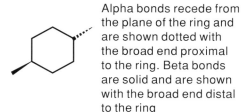

Alpha bonds recede from the plane of the ring and are shown dotted with the broad end proximal to the ring. Beta bonds are solid and are shown with the broad end distal to the ring

Interchange arrow (starting from the right)

Interchange arrow (starting from the left)

Flow charts

Flow charts are intended to show a sequence of events or the structure of an organisation. These charts may sometimes be enhanced by shadow effects but we feel this is more effective on slides than it is for publication, where decoration is best avoided. Boxes at the same level of importance should be kept the same size.

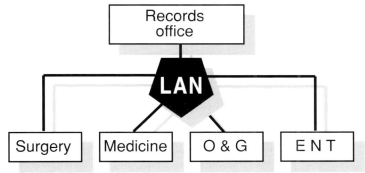

The shadow is made by duplicating the drawing, filling and stroking with grey then sending it to the back, the work of a few seconds

Decision charts

There must be a clear distinction between positive and negative pathways. We suggest that the positive pathway should be emphasised. It is sometimes useful to stress the start and conclusion.

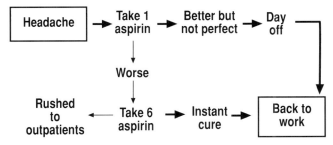

The non-designed graph

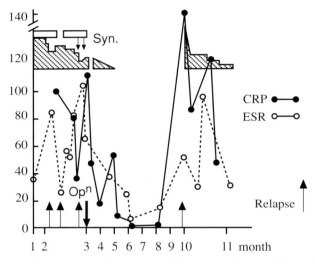

Miss X aged 14yrs. Pan-colonic Crohn's Dis.
CRP μg/ml.
ESR mm/hr.

This graph was intended for publication. It would not have passed editorial scrutiny for the following reasons:

1   It is generally confusing.

2   Although CRP and ESR may use the same digital scale values, it is never a good idea to superimpose two values that are measured in different units on the same graph.

3   Self-invented abbreviations have been used: eg. 'syn.' for synacthen, 'Op^n' for operation, Dis for disease and hr instead of h for hour.

4   Arrows denote direction or movement and should not perform meaningless functions.

5   Drug therapy has been drawn in a confusing manner, overlapping the graph line.

6   The legend has been placed in such a position that it will inevitably reduce the overall size of the data on the printed page. Is it necessary anyway?

7   Scale index marks (tick marks) have been drawn facing inwards. This is always a bad practice.

8   There are unaccountable differences in the unit length of the X-axis scale.

9   Scales are drawn beyond the last tick mark, creating an untidy appearance.

This case is fairly typical of many clinical situations. The doctor wanted to publish an interesting case and was undeterred by the fact that the clinical data were incomplete. The paper was accepted eventually, not only because of the medical issues involved, but also because the material was finally presented in a clear and honest manner.

The same data designed for acceptance

The graph below shows the same data but organised, simplified and using correct SI units. The anomalies in the X-axis scale have been drawn in a dotted line, and these were explained in the text. The narrow column has been maintained. This suits most journal pages and it meant that the original artwork did not require much reduction to fit the column width.

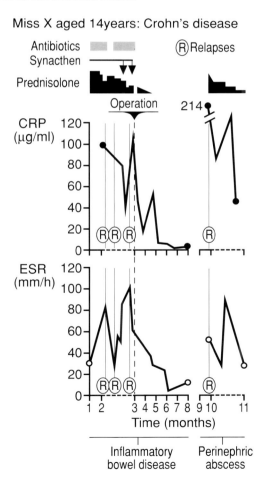

The anatomy of a good graph

The data will be used as a 35mm slide. The graph has been 'stretched' to the correct proportion

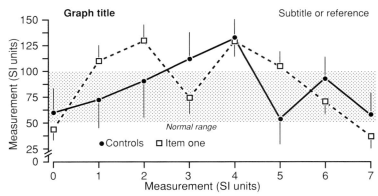

The basic rules

2:3 unit format for 35mm slides

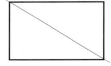

3:4 unit format for ciné or video

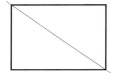

1:1 (or 2:3) for OHP

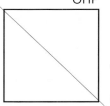

- Outward facing 'tick' marks prevent scales clashing with data near them.

- All major elements in the data are separated from the background by white areas around them–plotted points for example. This is so easy to achieve using computers and is so difficult with pen and ink.

- 'Controls' are shown boldest.

- Because the Y-axis does not start at zero, a break is shown.

- Standard error bars may sometimes be simplified and drawn in one direction to avoid overlaps.

- Always show normality. The normal range is clearly indicated.

- Always use SI units, never self-invented symbols.

- The size of lettering must suit the function of the illustration.

- Set the proportions of the overall shape to fill the area dictated by the function. Use a rectangle 2:3 (A4) for slides, a square (25 x 25cm or 10 x 10in) or rectangle 2:3 (A4) for OHP, and a rectangle 3:4 for ciné film, video, or presentation via 'Barco™' or similar unit.

- Avoid overlapping any symbol, text or part of the drawing with other parts.

- If leader lines are used, outline one side in white. This should always be the 'upper' side.

- Use one font if possible, varying the size if necessary.

× +
▫ ◉

1 litre not 1l
0° not O°

Note: Avoid the symbols shown on the right. They either print poorly or are ambiguous. Spell out 'litres' instead of using the abbreviation 'l'. As you can see here, the l and the 1 are hard to distinguish. Use zero and not capital O for numerals.

Summary

Setting up a graph style to use as a template for all future graphs is a great timesaver. Remember to stretch or shrink the graph to suit the format of presentation, filling the area with data not empty space. If submitting for journal publication, read the rules carefully. Some journals do not require you to include lettering. Some journals redraw the entire graph. Always use recognised abbreviations; be careful to spell these out if there is any likelihood of confusion. It isn't necessary to buy a separate graphing program for standard errors if you don't use these often.

ARTWORK FOR
OVERHEAD PROJECTION

9

Overhead projection is suitable for small audiences and those unhappy situations when not enough time has been allowed for the preparation of slides. OHP can be a very effective communication tool, provided that its limitations are understood. OHP encourages audience participation because of its informality. Basic techniques are discussed.

Designing for the overhead projector

Overhead projection is an extension of the classroom blackboard but is much more versatile. The size of the OHP projection screen is limited (on average about 2 x 2m or 6 x 6ft) and it is therefore suitable only for teaching small groups. It is important to format data specifically for this means of presentation and not merely photcopy existing journal or book texts.

The advantages of OHP can be summed up as:

- The lecturer faces the audience.
- Informality.
- The audience is more likely to participate.
- Materials are inexpensive. OHP lends itself to DIY.
- Information can be assembled and dismantled in a variety of sequences.
- A limited form of animation is possible.
- Hand-drawn 'instant' information can be added at any time during the presentation. This allows you to respond to audience participation.
- Lecture rooms do not need to be completely darkened.

There may be at
least one person
in the audience
whose view is
masked

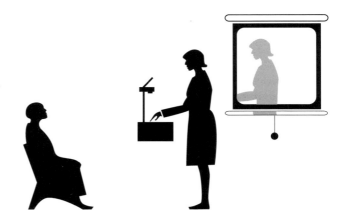

There are some disadvantages to the use of OHP that are often overlooked:

- Because the medium is often used in an informal manner, the way the seating is arranged can affect how much of the screen the audience will see. Their view can sometimes be blocked by the lecturer or by the projector head. Therefore the lower third of the projection area is not a good place to put vital information.

- Because OHP is an apparently 'casual' form of presentation, data are often prepared carelessly at the last minute and illegible transparencies are commonplace. The computer makes the preparation of artwork easy and this means that you can avoid handwritten OHP presentations.

Seating plan to
avoid masking the
screen

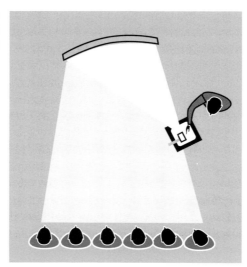

To avoid the problem of masking the view of the audience, the height of the bottom of the screen should be about 1.6m (5ft 6in) from the floor. But the best solution is to use a properly designed OHP screen (shallow convex shape) and arrange the room so that distortions caused by projecting at angles are reduced to a minimum, and the presenter is off-set to one side

When preparing artwork for OHP presentations, use the table on page 45. This will ensure the legibility of written data. It is vital to use heat-resistant transparencies, specially made for photocopiers or laserprinters, if expensive damage to your equipment is to be avoided.

Four basic techniques

We would always advocate the use of OHP card frames. These are available to support both A4 and 25 x 25cm (10 x 10in) formats. Transparency film is very slippery and easy to drop and can thus get scratched or otherwise damaged. Card frames allow you to organise and store OHP film in an efficient manner. The frames themselves can be used for your own notes and reminders as you present your talk, and additional transparencies can be attached to any of the four sides.

The use of additional transparencies attached to a card frame provides a maximum of five pictures for any one frame. These can be shown in sequence, building up the data in comfortable stages.

Four-sheet flip build-up

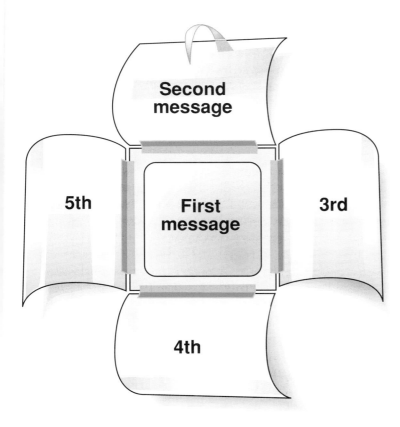

Stage by stage revealing, good for diagrams The example below shows an ideal way of revealing groups of data that are related. It is particularly useful for showing parts of a diagram, allowing you to talk about each part before revealing the whole.

Reveal first   Reveal second

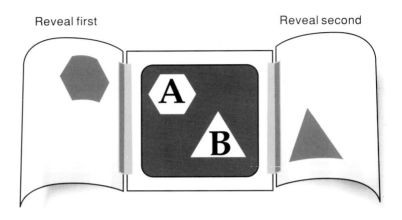

Point by point revealing, good for text

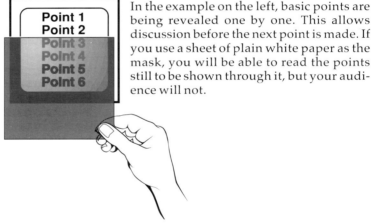

In the example on the left, basic points are being revealed one by one. This allows discussion before the next point is made. If you use a sheet of plain white paper as the mask, you will be able to read the points still to be shown through it, but your audience will not.

Simple animation

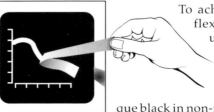

To achieve simple animation, flexible, low-tack tape is used to reveal a hidden object quite slowly. The artwork is printed in reverse (clear film where the image is and opaque black in non-image areas). Not all tape is flexible enough to cope with very tight curves. You will have to experiment.

Some useful tips

In some circumstances there may be glare from the screen, and *Avoiding glare* this may not help the legibility of serifed letterforms. Glare can be reduced by laying a lightly tinted transparent colour on the projector. This is advisable for monochrome OHP transparencies only, as it would otherwise affect the colours being projected. The best colour for a tinted glare-reducing film is yellow, as this helps to enhance the contrast of projected images without reducing light output very much.

Drawing and illustration programs that use vector mapping or *Using drawing* pathway mapping are ideal for producing OHP material. The *and illustration* complete 'story' can be drawn and then, using the fact that the *programs* image consists of a number of separate 'objects', each object can be put onto a different transparency for re-assembly during the lecture.

Colours work best in overhead projection if fully saturated. Col- *Colour* ours that look too rich on the film itself may project very well. Pale colours may project as anaemic or white. This is because there is always an element of desaturation via the ambient light in the room. Always use colour functionally and not decoratively.

All presentations are improved if some time is given to the plan- *Planning your* ning stages. We advise using a storyboard for getting your *presentation* thoughts in order and for sketching ideas for illustrations.

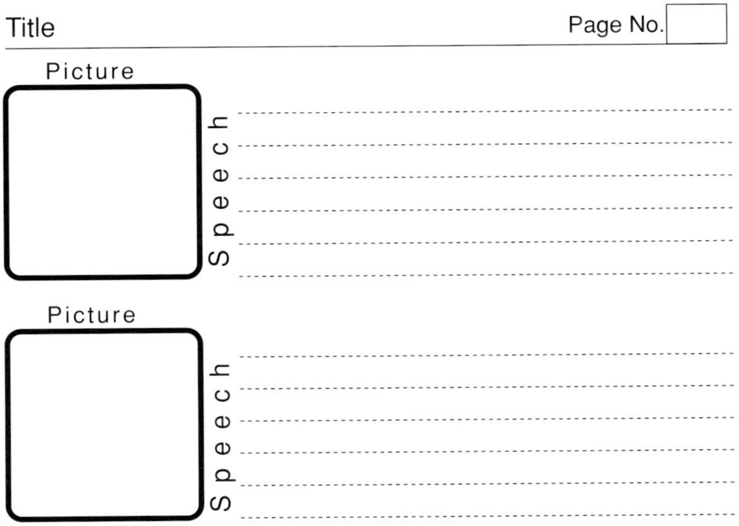

Title		Page No.	A storyboard planning sheet

Picture

Speech

Picture

Speech

A storyboard such as the one shown above can be set up in any wordprocessing or drawing/illustration package, and provides about four units per A4 page. If you write about 40 words these will take about 20 seconds to present — if you take it nice and easy.

Checklist

- Use a mount to help protect your work. Mounts usually have a choice of window sizes, either 25 x 25cm (10 x 10in) or A4. Some mounts can be converted to the larger size by punching out the upper and lower panels.

- Design your information with the correct format in mind. 25 x 25cm is square; A4 is oblong.

- Leave a 25mm (1in) margin all round to allow for inefficient projection and also so that there is room to put tape when fixing a transparency to the mount.

- Use a sans serif letter style, in not less than 18pt if there is likely to be a large audience or if you are uncertain of ambient lighting conditions.

- The lines used for drawing should not be thinner than 0.5mm.

- Avoid using handwriting.

- If you are using colours, use them to connect related items, not just for decoration. Use strong colours.

- Rehearse your presentation, particularly if you are using a variety of presentation techniques. This will help the action to go smoothly.

- *Always* use heat resistant transparency sheets, designated for photocopying or laserprinting.

Summary

OHP presentation should not be taken casually. Avoid using handwriting if you can. Now that computers are available they should be used to create good legible lettering and diagrams. Use a storyboard at the planning stage. Not only does this help you to organise pictures with text, it can also help you to pace your presentation so that it moves comfortably. Make sure that you use simple letterforms, preferably sans serif, and a bold style if lighting conditions are likely to be poor.

ARTWORK FOR POSTERS

10

Poster presentations are advertisements for your work and for your department .They require good planning, the mere enlargement of a short report will never be successful. You are in competition with your colleagues, and have to sell your ideas to an audience whose time may be severely limited. What is the most economical way of spending time and other resources to produce something which often does not have a long life span? Standards of legibility and simple production methods are discussed.

Designing for posters

The presenters of scientific posters are in a highly competitive environment, with very little time to 'sell' themselves and their ideas. The enlargement of bits and pieces from recent publications is no way to advertise your work. It is important to present the essential message boldly using some of the propaganda techniques associated with advertising, simplifying the message to basics and keeping the detail for a handout.

It is an advantage to make your poster template in a drawing program. This will allow you to set type in columns and to have access to drawing features such as lines, boxes, tones and colours. We have found that drawing programs give more flexibility than either wordprocessing or page make-up programs. Once a style has been set it can be used on other occasions. *What program?*

A two-stage approach is often used, with the text going initially into a wordprocessing format, then being imported into a draw program for enhancements. We advocate the use of integrated programs, such as ClarisWorks™, which offer most of what you need for posters combined into one. Microsoft Word™ has the advantage of also including an equation editor and limited graphing features, but it is less able to cope with drawings.

Planning Start planning by using a storyboard such as we advocate for slides and OHP presentations. Posters usually need to be a severe précis of your subject. Make it sound exciting. An essential part of a good poster presentation is the handout that should accompany it. The handout can give all the details you had to leave out, as well as providing contact addresses and additional references.

Economics The economics of poster production have to be considered: How can we make the time spent in manufacture and the cost involved worth it? Firstly, let's remember that computers, used efficiently, save much of the labour time, particularly if you make several posters per year and set up a style sheet for their production. Secondly, consider how posters may be able to continue to work for you as demonstrations, to your colleagues and visitors, of the work that is being done by yourself or your department.

If you intend to use your poster again, it may make sense to go for a more sophisticated presentation. Posters can be produced in full colour by colour photocopying, dye sublimation and wax transfer four-colour printing, straight from computer disc in either Macintosh or IBM formats. These methods are no longer as expensive as they were. Local high street printshops will often advise about the most recent progress in low-cost colour printing.

Design It is essential to remember the following points when designing *principles* poster presentations:

- Posters need to be eye-catching and attractive so that people will stop and look at them.

- All lettering should be legible from at least 1m (3ft 3in). The standard viewing distance given by most organisers is about 1.5 metres. The formula given on page 45 will give you some idea of the correct text size for legibility.

- There should be a clear hierarchical structure to the information.

Two ways of dealing with information: the first is boring, the second more eye-catching

Introduction	Introduction
What did I do? How did I do it? What were the results? Are they significant? What do my peers think? What is the background and references? How long will it be before this work is recognised and I get the Nobel Prize? or the Victoria Cross for bravery in such a competitive field?	● What did I do? ● How did I do it? ● What were the results? ● Are they significant? ● What is the background and references?

- You must include illustrations. Enlarged text alone is unattractive and a bore.
- Colour increases attractiveness but should be used with discretion so as not to impair legibility.

The structure of information is typically as follows: ***Information structure***

- Title (Needs to be punchy and not too verbose, in the style of a newspaper headline. It should be legible from at least 4-5m (12-15ft))
- Authors (Titles, names, addresses)
- Introduction (What did I do?)
- Methods (How did I do it?)
- Results (Did it work ?)
- Conclusions (Is it significant for the future?)

Viewers at a poster meeting are often short of time and so will look at the conclusions first, in order to satisfy themselves that the subject and its treatment are what they are interested in. For this reason, conclusions should be short, sharp, boldly stated and thought provoking, and in larger type than the rest of the text.

Methods of manufacture

If you have access to a photocopier which will enlarge to A3, you ***Using the*** may be able to produce texts, graphs and drawings all together at ***photocopier*** a suitable scale on your computer. You will need to first print them out as A4 laserprints, then enlarge them to A3 via the photocopier. Alternatively you can produce the whole poster using many 'pages' on the computer, then the resulting A4 sheets can be trimmed and fixed edge to edge, like tiles, to form the finished poster.

Some drawing and illustration programs will allow you to produce tiled artwork in excess of 1 metre by 1 metre (3ft 3in x 3ft 3in), and this is one of the reasons why we advocate the use of drawing/illustration programs for poster production.

One of the main problems facing the poster presenter is how best ***Transportation*** to transport it to the venue, since posters often consist of several ***problems*** parts, most of which are fragile. Photographs may be separate, machine traces can be sensitive to scratching or bending, and there may be last minute material which will only be fixed on site.

Unless all your data are in one piece, such as one large photographic print, we cannot recommend rolling the sheets. Your rolled-up material may pass through extreme environmental changes, especially if you are travelling overseas by air. By the time you reach your destination, your poster can be in a sorry

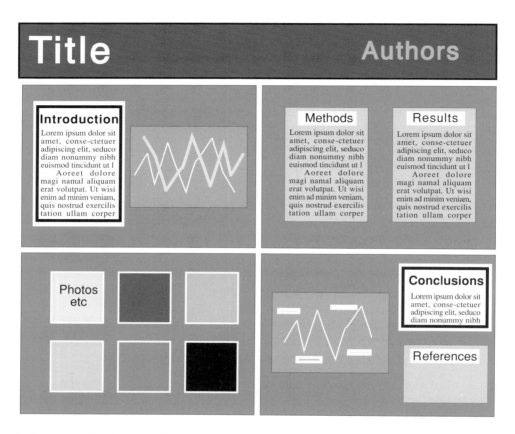

In the example above we have used four coloured A3 sheets of thin card in horizontal format. On these, A4 and A5 sheets of coloured text, photographs and drawings are mounted using spray glue. The title is also on card with enlarged and tiled lettering, first printed out on A4 and then cut to fit. The title board can be scored lightly on the back so that it folds, face to face, or it can be made from several pieces taped together at the back. The entire package size is no more than A3 (29.7 x 42cm or 11.75 x 16.5in). The overall size of the poster here is 60.9 x 84.0cm (2ft 6in x 2ft 8in), including 15cm (6in) for the vertical dimension of the title board

state. Photographs may have become unstuck and other sheets may be annoyingly unwilling to go flat again. You may be given very little time to mount your poster on arrival, and having to deal with problems of this nature when pressed for time can be very unnerving.

Advantages of a modular system The single large photographic print sounds ideal but is usually expensive. We advocate using a sheet of mounting card that will fit into a suitcase or can be wrapped and carried under the arm. For this reason we believe the A3 modular system to be the most practical. Using this modular technique your data can be printed on A4 sheets of coloured paper, these can be fixed to the card with spray glue, and the result can be effective and inexpensive.

The ideal lettering sizes for the various parts of a poster are given below and are intended for the method suggested above where an A4 sheet is enlarged by 141% to A3. The best way is to experiment with your own ideas and text styles, but do make sure that the data are legible from the distances advised by the organisers — usually not closer than one metre (3ft 3in). ***Recommended lettering sizes***

- Titles: 48pt Times Roman™ bold on a 54pt linefeed.
- Names: 24pt Helvetica™ regular italic on a 30pt linefeed.
- Addresses: 18pt Helvetica™ regular italic on a 22p linefeed.
- Subheadings: 24pt Helvetica™ bold on a 30pt linefeed.
- Text: Times Roman™ 18pt regular on a 22pt linefeed.

Before work begins, it is vital to find out whether the longest dimension of the allocated poster space is horizontal or vertical. Mistakes can be very untidy. ***Horizontal and vertical formats***

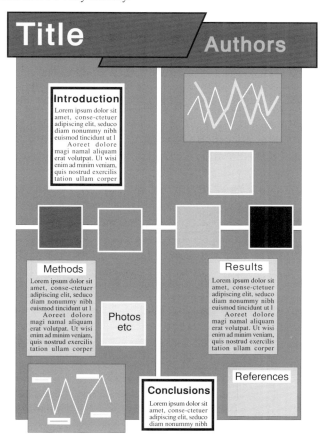

This is what can happen if you prepare a horizontal poster and have to fit it into a vertical space

Checklist

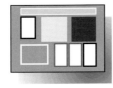

- Is the long axis of your allocated space vertically or horizontally orientated?
- What are the rules about lettering sizes?
- Will the organisers supply the artwork for the title board?
- What fixing methods are allowed or supplied by the organisers?
- How will you transport the poster? As flat sheets, or pre-mounted on boards, or as rolls? Rolls may present a fixing problem because of their tendency to wind up again.
- Is it possible that the poster will NOT become junk at the end of the show but be used as good departmental propaganda later? If so, design with more sophistication in mind, using better methods of production.

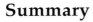

Summary

Never take the lazy option of merely enlarging recent publications. Computers have made it possible to design posters quickly and efficiently using good-looking graphics and legible lettering. The use of style sheets is recommended for situations where poster production is commonplace. There are some standard ways of presenting data and these should be followed. Use newspaper presentation as a model — aim to surprise your audience. Make an interesting précis of your subject, leaving the viewer wanting to know more. Provide an informative handout giving more detail, and don't forget to include contact addresses for further communication.

DESIGNING FOR PROJECTION: 35mm SLIDES AND CINÉ/VIDEO

11

Slides should require the presence of the lecturer to explain them. They need to illustrate *one* idea at a time. Enough slides should be made to cope with this. Use a storyboard to organise your presentation. Data on a slide should be designed to fit within the chosen slide format. Always rehearse your presentation and carefully check the legibility factors. Beware of the format difference between 35mm projection and ciné/video projection.

Planning a slide presentation

There should always be a partnership between the image on the screen, the lecturer and the audience. This interaction can be broken by illegible slides, or by an audience reading a slide while the lecturer boringly repeats the same words as if in a kindergarten. We suggest that the best way to use slides is to design their messages in a 'telegram' style. This means that the pictures or texts are not self explanatory but *require* the presence of the lecturer.

Pacing your presentation

Slides are simply pictures on a wall; they have little value unless they illustrate something. The gist of the message has to be immediately obvious, but the time given for absorbing the detail is determined by you, the presenter. Be kind to your audience and give them a chance. What is so familiar to you may be stranger-than-fiction to them. We suggest that there is an optimum time for a slide to be viewed before the next one appears. This is about seven seconds. We are not suggesting, though, that all slides should be seen for the same length of time. The pacing will need to vary, depending on the manner of presentation. For example, if there is audience participation, a slide may need to be on screen for longer. Changes of pace will also help to keep the audience's interest alive. A slide presentation is a theatrical performance, a one-person show, with the audience wanting to be delighted with what they are seeing.

Optimum time
on-screen

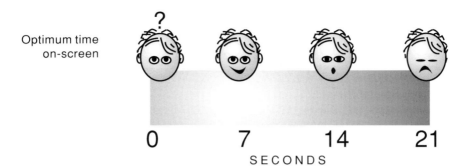

0   7   14   21

SECONDS

One idea per slide Never be afraid of using too many slides. One idea per slide is ideal. Think of the minds of the audience as being made of cotton wool (it's possible that some of them are); they will absorb your information more effectively if you pour it out slowly and in small amounts. Complex illustrations need breaking into simpler, more digestible chunks. Why show one slide when you can show five? The final slide and/or the first slide can both show the complex situation, if indeed you are offering one.

Using word slides Word slides are best used in one of two ways. They can either be used as signposts to remind the audience of the topics that you are dealing with, or they can be used to emphasise particular points. If they are used for emphasis, they should never make sense on their own. They are more effective (i.e. memorable) if they are like cryptograms, requiring the lecturer to decode them.

The storyboard We suggest the use of a storyboard as illustrated on page 127 (a reminder is shown here). A sketch for each picture is drawn in the box. If twenty to thirty words are written against it, it is probably time to think of another slide. Finally, the script planner becomes an aide mémoire for the actual presentation. It is important to bear in mind that writing for a slide presentation requires a simple and direct approach, whereas more detail can be included when writing for publication.

Title   Page No.

Picture

Speech

Designing for slides

Ideally, your slides should be consistent in their design. How- ***Consistent*** ever, this is often hard to achieve, particularly if your slides have ***presentations*** been assembled from several sources and over a long period. If the particular presentation is an important one and you want to create a good impression, it is sometimes worth re-making all the word slides so that they at least follow a common design style. This will help to create an overall impresssion of consistency.

35mm projection slides have a window for information which is ***Slide formats*** two units by three units The shape of the artwork must be the same. Fortunately an A4 sheet has roughly these proportions.

The best orientation for slides is with the long axis horizontal. This often projects better, especially in smaller lecture theatres where the ceiling height prevents the instal- lation of a large enough screen.

Standard 35mm slide format

The horizontal orientation is also needed for slide printing devices. If your data are unavoidably ver- tical then the best way to send this to a slide machine is to rotate the image through ninety degrees at the artwork stage. If your data happen to be unavoidably square, then you could choose a slide mount with a square window from the several formats available (examples are shown on page 138). The data will then project about 30% larger. But be warned, you have to use larger film for superslide windows, so it's worth it only if you have unavoidably complex data.

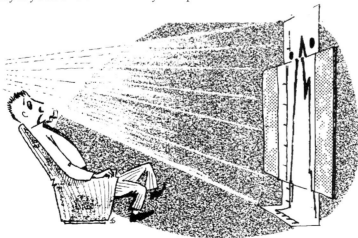

Vertical slide, horizontal screen

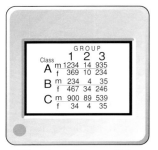

Standard 35mm slide

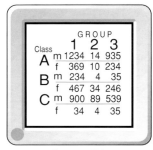

Superslide

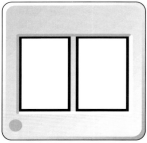

Pair 2:3 wimdows

Various slide window formats are shown here. If you have unavoidably square data it will project 1/3 larger on screen in a superslide mount, *but* this will require film larger than 35mm

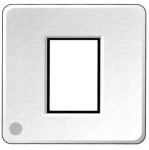

Small 2:3 window

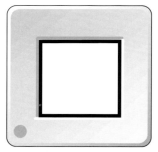

35mm film square window

Legibility We have already explained the principles of legibility of lettering as related to viewing distance (see page 45). Suffice it to say here that if the words on a slide are just legible with the naked eye as you hold the slide in your hand, then you are likely to have a slide that will be legible when projected.

We admit that on occasion there may be complex visual problems to be solved. Long lists of molecules or amino acid chains are examples of such problems. You may wish to show an entire sequence to illustrate certain links, similarities or differences at particular places in the chain or list. In this case, don't expect people to be able to see or read the precise details. You will have to employ the zoom-in, zoom-out technique to make all these levels of

information clear. So the first slide might show the entire construction and the next might be a close-up of an important detail.

We advise against using negative (white lines on a dark ground)   ***Use of 'negative'***
images for drawings. The world of objects that we normally see is   ***material***
not viewed in this mode. It is particularly confusing on slides.
And we might remember that if the audience is from a culture
other than our own, graphic representations may be harder to
grasp. Negative images add to this problem.

Where lettering is concerned, a negative slide, if properly designed, can look very good, but light images on negative slides
can appear to blur because of the spread of light. This often makes
thin lines difficult to see clearly, especially for those with impaired eyesight. It is therefore important to design negative slides
a little more boldly, with slightly more space between characters
and lines of text than would be the case for positive slides.

Preparing artwork for 35mm slides

Prepare a template that has on it a horizontal rectangle that is two   ***Templates***
units by three and fits comfortably within your computer screen.
This serves as a basis for all standard 35mm slides.

It is best not to put objects right up to the edges of this rectangle
because there is sometimes a slight mismatch between slide formats and projection equipment. As a guide, measure the diagonal
of the rectangle, deduct 15%, and draw a second rectangle, with
this shorter diagonal, inside the first. This is your artwork area.
All of your data must fit within it to guarantee projection of the

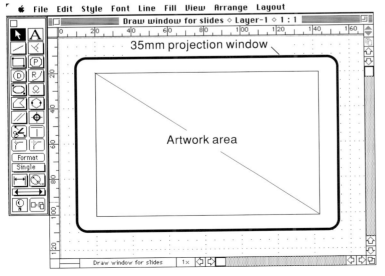

A standard 35mm
slide template as
it might appear on
the screen in a
drawing program

entire image. When the drawing is complete, the two rectangles can be discarded. Since all slides are naturally bounded by the slide window, we do not advocate using a drawn-in border.

Checking computer artwork Computerised slide production methods are normally fast *provided* nothing goes wrong, but there are many possible sources of error. For example, when you are preparing diagrams and have finished a drawing, zoom out to the smallest size and check that no image has inadvertently been put somewhere you did not expect. This is very easy to do when using the 'duplicate' feature in draw or illustration programs. In our example, the letter A has been mislaid and it was not visible in the normal view. If this goes to the slide printer it will result in very slow processing time and a minute image on the slide!

Finding stray items

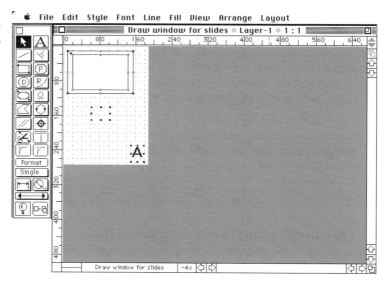

The same screen image as on the previous page but zoomed-out four times. We have used the command to 'select all'. It is vital to use this command as it will 'find' not only the visible letter 'A' but also invisible items such as the transparent box in the centre, now revealed by six small black squares. These unwanted images will cause havoc in the slide-making process if they are not removed

Check with the slide-making service Always check with the slide bureau or print service as to their precise requirements *before* you start designing. There are often limitations as to the fonts they have *and* they may need your data exported to disc in a particular manner. When designing your slides, play it safe and use only the regular 'system' fonts. Be kind to those who provide slide printing services and give them enough time, just in case things do not go according to plan.

Most slide-making services will mount your slides in glass mounts and we would support this as the glass protects slides from damage. However, if you use your slides in areas of high humidity such as the tropics, you may be advised to avoid glass since this creates a mini-greenhouse effect. Any material used in severe conditions will need to be inspected more often. If moulds start to grow, there are special film cleaners. Kodak have a leaflet dealing with the care of film materials in the tropics. *Care of film in the tropics*

Make sure that a spot has been placed on the lower lefthand corner of the slide when viewed from the front. This is the marker that tells you (or the projectionist) which way round to put your slides in the projector. It is particularly helpful when the orientation is not obvious. In the projector, slides must be right-reading but upside down (the spot will now be top right). *Marker spots on slides*

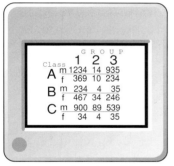
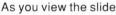

As you view the slide

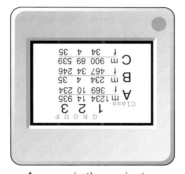

As seen in the projector

Rehearse your presentation

It is useful to rehearse in a 'real' situation. That is, find a lecture theatre and stand up and deliver your slides and talk, speaking more slowly and carefully than usual and timing the presentation carefully. This will increase your awareness, and you will be less likely to exceed your allotted time.

It is often a salutary experience to go to the back of a large lecture hall while someone else operates the projector for you. Sit down and think of yourself as a person only slightly familiar with your subject (always hard to do). View your own slides with dispassionate criticism. You may be surprised at what you see, but do please learn from it for the sake of your audience. Use your colleagues to help check your presentation — their opinions may be very helpful. *Check your slides*

It is important to avoid the tendency to treat the screen as a blackboard and to turn towards it in order to confirm that the picture is the one you think it is. This bad habit weakens your presentation *The screen is not a blackboard* and at the same time makes what you are saying harder to hear. It is possible to use a cheap suction-based driving mirror on the rostrum. This helps confirm the image on the screen without turning your head. The mirror must be convex and you will probably have to supply it. This is something that rostrum designers have not yet thought of.

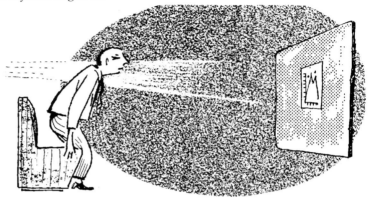

Try looking at your own slides from the back of a large lecture hall!

Artwork for ciné or video projection

The rules for legibility that we have already mentioned also apply to ciné or video projection. When working direct from the computer screen, the screen itself becomes your artwork area.

There is one essential difference, however. The shape of the usable area is no longer two units by three but three units by four. This format is also used when preparing artwork for cinematography. If this format is not observed you risk losing data at the edges of the screen. If your artwork is in colour, fully saturated colours should be used and the room must be fully darkened to take account of the poorer light emission from video projectors than from slide projectors.

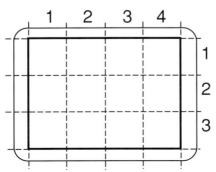

The 3:4 ciné/video format is much 'squarer' than the 2:3 format for 35mm slide. Be prepared to increase lettering sizes. A test will indicate whether this is needed

Projection problems

The distances and viewing angles from which the audience views slides are intimately woven into the legibility of projected data. We mention a few of the basic problems here in order to explain why we stress that the size of projected lettering should never go below our minimum recommendations.

We assume that the lecture theatre or seminar room is properly blacked out. Too much ambient light will destroy any projected colours. Adequate ventilation is often hard to reconcile with blackout, but the audience will go to sleep if they don't get enough air.

The optimum audience distance from any screen is somewhere between two and six screen diagonals. At less than two screen diagonals the images are likely to appear rough or out of focus. Beyond six diagonals, lettering will rapidly become too small to read.

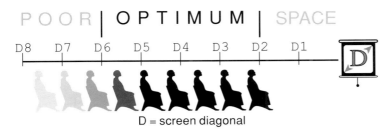

D = screen diagonal

The optimum viewing angle is thirty degrees to the right and left of the centre line. The audience sitting at the ends of the rows will have a seriously impaired view if their viewing angle reaches forty five degrees.

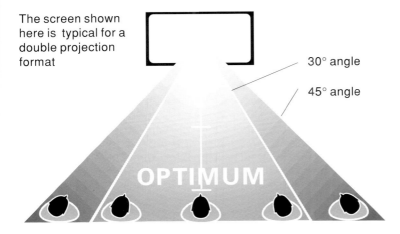

The screen shown here is typical for a double projection format

30° angle

45° angle

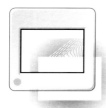

Checklist

- What are the requirements of your slide-making service? Do they expect your material to be printed to disc in a particular manner? What are their font requirements?

- Glass mounts keep your slides cleaner.

- Use a storyboard to plan your presentation.

- Prepare a template for designing standard 35mm slides. Remember, the area for artwork is two units by three units.

- Use colour as a method of coding related parts, not just for decoration.

- Search for stray unwanted items on your artwork before sending discs to the slide-printer.

- Rehearse your presentation and time the duration of your speech. Use the assistance of colleagues, especially for important meetings.

- Prepare a handout if you think this will be useful for the audience. It can elaborate on details and provide contact addresses, references etc..

- Use a convex driving mirror with a suction base if you feel it would help prevent you turning your head away from the audience.

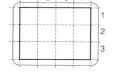

- If the data are for ciné or video projection, then the area for design is three units by four.

- If you possibly can, try out some sample illustrations on the video system you will be using. Video systems can vary in their efficiency. If in doubt, increase lettering sizes and their contrast against the background colour to ensure legibility.

Summary

Slides have their limitations. Not all data are suitable for this mode of presentation. Deliver one idea per slide, but use enough slides to do the job. Artwork should be prepared within a template and the correct size of lettering used. Use word slides sparingly. Rehearsals build confidence and will help you to keep to your allotted time. If you are using ciné or video projection, increased lettering size and contrast with the background might be needed, and it will be essential to design within a space three units by four.

PREPARING MANUSCRIPTS FOR CAMERA-READY COPY OR DISC-TO-IMAGESETTER & POSTING YOUR ARTWORK

12

Make sure that the content of your document is organised logically. Initially keep the layout and typography as simple as possible. Orchestrate only after you have the tune. Evolve a system of stages and apply the full design near the last stage. Always contact the printing house or publisher at an early stage so that you can keep in step with their procedures. We suggest a basic plan. Hardcopy artwork has its own problems.

Content planning

The first task is to organise the content of your text. It should have a beginning, a middle and an end, and should be divided into a suitable number of chapters, sections and subsections. With wordprocessing techniques it doesn't matter where you begin writing, but it will save time if you draw up a skeleton list of main headings before you begin and than add flesh to the bones. You should also bear in mind the possibility of using listed points where they would be clearer than continuous text, and write accordingly. When you have finished writing you should check that your headings form a logical structure and that you have treated similar kinds of information consistently throughout. If your writing is not logical and consistent, it will be impossible to give it a clear visual structure by means of typography and layout. Some useful books on writing are listed on page 185 under 'Further reading'.

Early stages in wordprocessing

Regardless of how you intend to produce your final output, if you are new to wordprocessing you should keep your layout as simple as possible until you are satisfied with the content of your text. It is unnecessary at the beginning to have a clear idea about the design of your document. This can be dealt with much later.

One of the major advantages of electronic imagery is the flexibility you have to alter and edit material throughout the process of its generation. This flexibility is destroyed if preconceptions about design are allowed to fix all movement at an early stage. So don't try to orchestrate before you have the tune. Effort and therefore time will be wasted. Secretaries with a 'traditional' typing background often find the 'undesigned' initial-stage document difficult to accept, but it is vital that it should be typed in this way.

The following points summarise what we have found to be the best procedure in the early stages of wordprocessing.

- Remember that there is an essential difference between typefaces (fonts) used for presentation on the computer screen and fonts resident in the printer (see page 14). Start by wordprocessing in a typeface resident in your printer and use whatever 'default' spacing your particular program favours. Once you are familiar with the difference between printer and screen fonts, you may prefer to use a screen font (such as Geneva) when you are typing or editing your text. This will make the text easier to read on the screen. You can then convert the entire text to printer fonts at the design and layout stage.

- Always set the text to a flush-left margin. In particular, never justify (set parallel margins) to text that will later be imported into a page make-up program.

- It is best to insert only *essential* carriage returns, i.e. one return at the end of each paragraph.

- Insert headings and subheadings as if they were new paragraphs.

- If you have been asked to produce a 'double spaced' manuscript, don't do this by typing in carriage returns. Your wordprocessing program will offer you a range of options for line spacing and it is very easy to change the spacing at any stage.

- It can be a serious disadvantage to start using indents and tabulation too soon. You may have to go back and alter them all if you change your mind about the structure of the document as you write, and they can cause problems if you want to import the text into a page make-up program at a later stage.

- Never use the underline. There are professional typographic tricks to emphasise words, as explained in Chapter 5.

- Never type two or more spaces after a full stop or any other punctuation mark. This habit is a hangover from the typewriter. The letter and word spacing in typeset text is much more sophisticated, so extra spaces are unnecessary. They will merely create white 'holes' in the text which will distract the reader's attention. They can also introduce unwanted digital codes, making it very difficult to translate between machines or programs later.

- Do not add spaces inside parentheses (round brackets).
- If it is important to distinguish between the numeral '1' and the letter 'l', and between the letter 'O' and zero, make sure that you type the correct character, and choose a typeface where these differences exist.
- Always maintain a *copy* of the text in this simple format, just in case you or someone else needs it later. It can be difficult to undo complex typographical layouts.

Nearly all the major wordprocessing packages have a word count provision should you find it necessary to keep the length of a document in mind.

Wordprocessed text as final output

Once the text is written, checked and corrected, start formatting and designing the final version. This is now the stage to make final decisions about such matters as the typeface, type size, line length, number of columns, justification and line spacing. Some of these decisions will depend on such things as the binding method and margins, as discussed in Chapter 4. You will also need to decide on the treatment of headings, paragraphs, listed points, tables, and so on. Many writing programs allow you to set up 'styles' for each kind of text you insert. Thus you can create a style for headings, another style for text and so on. It is therefore possible to create the pattern for the final orchestration and then make the tune fit into it.

Wordprocessing as a prelude to page make-up

If you are later going to set your text through a page make-up program, your wordprocessed text should be in the simple format described above and in one column only. It is usually a positive disadvantage to introduce complex variations in typography and spacing at the wordprocessing stage. This advice is given because the capability of import/export software varies in sophistication. Complex levels of indentation and different ways of dealing with carriage returns, margin or column settings can play havoc with the original wordprocessed layout. If you want to retain the tabulation settings of your wordprocessed text when importing this into a page make-up program, the length of line (measure) of your wordprocessed text must be less than the measure of the final page.

Page make-up

The function of the document now becomes important. It is necessary to decide the size of page, the margins and column widths. You cannot do this until you know how the document will be printed and bound. Will there be headers and/or footers, footnotes and page numbers? What is the most economical or most good looking type face? How will titles, headings and subheadings be dealt with? Page make-up programs allow you to set up style sheets for all typographic elements of the document, for example, headings, main text, captions and so on. It is very important to do this at an early stage. Modifying style sheets later will give rise to extra time-consuming work.

The type of paper to be used will affect the optimum choice of resolution of any photographs and the manual will provide information about resolution for various printing technologies. But the most important advice of all is to discuss the entire project with the printshop or publisher *before* starting.

Tables

Tables are now amongst the easiest things to set instead of being the very real problem they used to be. They may be imported directly from a spreadsheet or from database software, they may be imported from a drawing program, or they may have been prepared in the same wordprocessing program that has been used for the text. Microsoft Word™ and ClarisWorks™ can both set up tables within, but unconnected with, the general text by embedding a spreadsheet within it. This allows for the setting-up of multiple columns and the editing of any numerals or texts independently within or across columns without resetting or interfering with any other parts of the general text. Make sure you understand and use the appropriate tabs for the kind of data you are dealing with. There is, for example, a tab which centres columns of numerals under the decimal point.

If you have to set a large table, it can be very useful to use a much smaller typeface than that used in the general text. This will enable you to see the whole table on the screen so that you can judge the correct column spacing. You can always increase the type size later by re-sizing the whole table as a unit.

Illustrations: drawings or photographs

Drawings or photographs can be imported from other programs. If you are using a do-it-all program (such as ClarisWorks™) for wordprocessing, you will be able to create drawings within the same program. However, if you intend to produce the final result via a page make-up program, don't include the illustrations in the wordprocessed version; it is better to keep them separate. The page make-up program will tell you how pictures should be imported. It is usually possible to re-size them to fit any given space once they are imported.

Planning for printing

If you are preparing a document for use as camera-ready copy (CRC) or to send to an imagesetter at a commercial printing house, you will need to observe certain rules. Camera-ready copy means that the work will be photographed onto a printing surface of some kind and the copies will usually be made by offset lithography. This means that the best quality 'originals' will have to be used; second generation prints such as those made on a photocopier will not produce such good results. Similarly, work for reproduction by an imagesetter will have to be presented on disc, with absolutely no errors, since the proofreading stage is usually over when discs go direct to imagesetters. A good quality proof will be essential at some point so that document length, style, grammar, spelling and layout can all be checked by the interested parties. A good deal of thought therefore needs to go into planning documents for reproduction systems, but this can proceed from the simple to the complex in an orderly manner, as we have described above.

Resolution = quality

It is important to remember that the resolution or sharpness of the text and illustrations is entirely 'output device dependent' and is described in terms of dots per inch (dpi). The resolution of digital data is perfect, but as displayed on your screen it may only appear at a resolution of about 72dpi, whereas the same data printed via a Linotron imagesetter could appear at 2540dpi. A black line printed at 72-80dpi will appear very coarse and rough; at 300dpi, which is the low end of laserprinting, dots may be just discernable to the human eye; but at 2540dpi the dots are way beyond the resolution capabilities of the unaided human eye, so every drawing will look exceptionally smooth. Resolution as high as 2540dpi is hardly needed except for fine photographic images to be printed on top quality paper. For black and white drawings, 1270dpi is sufficient for top quality images.

Camera-ready copy: getting the best from laserprinters

If the intention is to produce work for camera-ready copy, then it **Paper** can be very important to do the final laserprint onto matt or semi-matt coated paper. These papers are kaolin coated and give the best smooth edges to the printed image. Do not use glossy papers. The image is less likely to fuse onto the paper and the shine can be a serious disadvantage in the subsequent photography. Always check with the production manager or editor before doing the final printing for CRC.

Page setup   Different printing devices have different ways of handling the page area, so before you print any document make sure that the page setup is correct for the device you are using. For example, if you print a draft on a non-laserprinter and then print the final version on a laserprinter without checking the page setup, you may find that the line breaks and page breaks have changed. This may mean that parts of the text that should remain together are now split across two pages.

Lettering quality   Obtaining high quality lettering is one of the major problems facing those who produce their own artwork for teaching and for publication. Publishers' requirements are usually very rigorous and should be adhered to if rejection of papers is to be avoided. Fortunately, laserprinters working at 300dpi resolution may be just acceptable for publication, provided the toner cartridge is in good condition and the correct grade of paper is used (see above). Printers offering 600dpi are much better of course and can imitate the high quality letterforms normally associated with 'professional' printing establishments.

Fonts   Always make sure you use fonts that are available on your intended printing device. Fonts such as Geneva, New York, Monaco and Chicago have been designed to be legible at the low resolution of the computer screen, but there are no printing device equivalents (see page 14).

Certain font names are the copyright of the original type manufacturers, and companies like Apple have licences allowing them to use these names. Times Roman™, Helvetica™, Bookman™, New Century Schoolbook™, Avant Garde™, Symbol™ and Courier™, for example, are all typefaces licensed to Apple and are accurately matched by Apple laserprinters. Beware of laserprinters that have fonts with similar names such as T Roman, TR or Times. They are not equivalents, and if you change from one laserprinter to another or from a laserprinter with non-standard fonts to an imagesetter, you may find that your line breaks and page breaks have changed.

Preparation for commercial printing

Many journals now expect to print direct from your computer disc. This is done in a variety of ways depending on the requirements of the publisher. Your disc may go directly to the editor who will put it on his or her screen for comparison with the hardcopy and for editing to suit the publisher's house style. Or the disc may go straight to the imagesetter — not a person but a printing device — where it will be set exactly as it is. It is important to find out precisely what the requirements of the printing house are before sending discs. Much time is wasted in these establishments trying to convert work unsuited to a particular press's methods. One of the main causes of delay is when the customer fails to supply both the printer fonts and the equivalent screen fonts that have been used in the document. It is always important to ask about the fonts the printing house has available.

Your printing house may require you to deliver your work with crop and registration marks. These help the printer to align and cut pages properly. The marks are inserted on request in page make-up programs. You will not be able to proof crop marks for an A4 page on an A4 printer, but they will be there for the commercial printer to see. The crop mark facility may be lacking in wordprocessing programs. In this case you may have to prepare a style sheet or template first, using the drawing mode.

Care of artwork

Our illustrations show typical cases of damage to hardcopy artwork. A cover sheet should always be put over work and lightly fastened to the back. The sheet may require removal later, depending on how the work is to be reproduced. Electronic artwork is, of course, not quite so prone to the risks associated with physical materials (except perhaps magnetism). The cover sheet is there for the editor to use for notes etc. and to protect against the inevitable coffee cup stains.

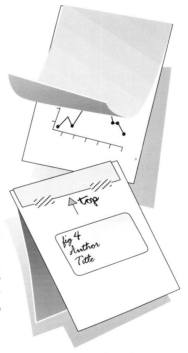

Paperclips do untold damage during postal delivery. Never use any hard object in contact with photographs, either from the back or front. The indentations are very time consuming and expensive to eliminate.

It is usual to affix a label on the back of hardcopy artwork and photographs, making sure that an arrow indicates the top

We recommend packing artwork and photographs of differing sizes in close fitting envelopes and taping these to a slightly over-size piece of card. This prevents them from sliding over each other in the post.

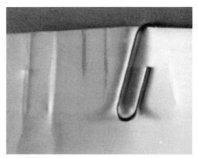

Damage caused in the post
by paperclips

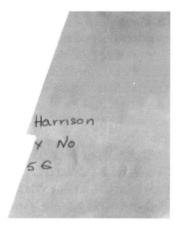

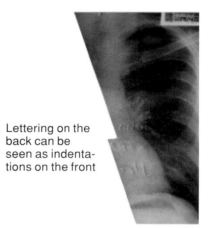

Lettering on the back can be seen as indentations on the front

Summary

Check that the content of your document is logically organised. Make your initial layout very simple. In wordprocessing, design effort should be reserved for the end of the cycle. In page make-up, design should be set up very carefully at the beginning. Page make-up usually requires detailed discussion with a publisher or printshop *before* any work is done. Make sure you understand that printer fonts are different from screen fonts.When sending text-on-disc to publishers you *must* work to their specifications. Be aware of the dangers of using paperclips in the post, and don't mark up photographs with anything hard.

WORKING COMFORT, HEALTH AND INSURANCE

13

We often neglect the obvious and simple precautions that we can take to protect both our health and that of the equipment and data we are working with. Some obvious environmental conditions are considered and pointers offered for controlling or improving them. Various hazards are discussed: theft, virus infection, environmental risks and data loss. What are the insurance options?

Working comfort

If you are likely to be using your computer for extended periods, it is important to pay attention to your working environment. A badly planned working area can damage your health, as well as reducing your efficiency.

Working space

Your working surface should be deep enough to enable you to place the computer screen directly in front of you at a comfortable distance. Many people find that a viewing distance of about 60cm (24in) is ideal, but you will need to test this for yourself. This means that your work surface will need to have a depth of 75-90cm (30-36in), depending on the depth of your VDU. You will then be able to place the keyboard between you and the screen.

The screen should be approximately at or just below eye level. You may like to consider using a small plinth or adjustable support if the screen seems too low.

You will also need adequate space on either side of the keyboard to place the papers and books (perhaps even a manual or two!) that you need to refer to as you work. The various adjustable document holders on the market enable you to position documents at about the same level and angle as the screen so that reference back and forth is made easier. Some stands incorporate a moveable horizontal guide, which is invaluable if you are copy-typing.

Posture A comfortable chair with adjustable support for the lumbar region of the back is essential. If your chair does not provide adequate back support, you will very soon begin to suffer with backache. The height of the seat must also be adjustable. You should set the height so that your forearms are approximately horizontal as you type and your feet rest comfortably on the floor. It is important that your arms should be in the correct position, and if this means that your feet dangle uncomfortably you will need to use a footrest of some kind. If you are not seated at the correct height in relation to the keyboard, you will probably find that your shoulders and neck begin to ache, and possibly your head too.

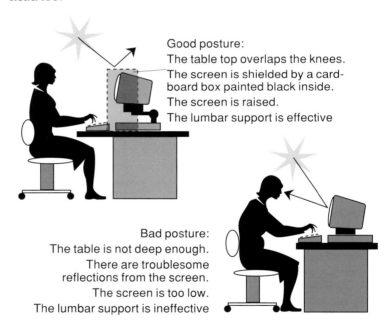

Good posture:
The table top overlaps the knees.
The screen is shielded by a cardboard box painted black inside.
The screen is raised.
The lumbar support is effective

Bad posture:
The table is not deep enough.
There are troublesome reflections from the screen.
The screen is too low.
The lumbar support is ineffective

Some computer screens can be switched from positive (i.e. a dark image on a light background) to negative (a light image on a dark background). We strongly advise the use of positive screens.

Negative screens have several disadvantages:

• The image on the screen bears little relation to the appearance of the final printout.

• Bright characters glowing against a dark screen will appear to spread and fill, thus decreasing legibility.

• Troublesome reflections are difficult to avoid.

- Constantly referring back and forth from a light sheet of paper to a dark screen may be tiring.

Positive screens have the following advantages:

- They give a much more accurate impression of what the image will look like when it is printed.

- The characters will not appear to spread in the same way as on a negative screen, so legibility is improved.

- Reflections are much less troublesome.

- The contrast when referring back and forth from paper to screen is less extreme and likely to be less tiring.

If you find the brightness of a positive screen tiring, this can usually be adjusted to suit your personal preferences.

Glare filters

There are two sorts of anti-reflection filters. The cheaper ones consist of a fine mesh, while the more expensive ones are polarising. Some people find that the cheaper filters increase eye strain rather than reducing it. This may be because the mesh creates a fuzzy image which the eyes are constantly trying to bring into sharp focus. We would argue that it is far better to reposition the computer or rearrange the room lighting than to put your sight at risk by using any methods that degrade the screen image.

Lighting

Your computer should ideally be placed in a room with diffuse lighting to reduce reflections on the screen. It is important to prevent strong light from falling directly on the screen as this will reduce contrast and hence legibility.

Spectacle wearers

If you normally wear spectacles for reading, you may find that you need a special pair for reading from the screen. Your normal reading glasses are intended for a reading distance of 40cm (16in) or so, and they may not give a satisfactory image of the screen at 60-75cm (24-30in). It is possible to obtain spectacles coated with an ultraviolet filter. Incorrect spectacles for computer work are probably the most common cause of headaches, since a combination of factors are at work. The very act of straining to get the screen properly in focus will cause you to crane your neck forward. It is this poor posture that is responsible for much long term discomfort.

Health

Radiation

The question of whether radiation from the screen is likely to be a health hazard is a controversial one, though there seems to be some agreement that pregnant women should avoid working with VDUs on a regular basis. If you would like more information, contact:

Health and Safety Executive
Regina House
259-269 Old Marylebone Road
London NW1 5RR
Telephone 071 723 1262

RSI By far the most common health hazards are associated with bad
posture and not resting enough or at regular intervals. The fa-
mous RSI (repetitive strain injury) is largely self inflicted — there
is no need for it. Computers are addictive to some people and to
others they are a tyrannical oppressor. Both make the user spend
more time working with them than is reasonable. The application
of common sense would do much to alleviate all the more common physical complaints. If you suffer from aches and pains or
eye strain of any kind, before rushing off to your doctor refer to
our notes on posture and the use of correctly adjusted glasses (if
you wear them).

The general environment

Badly sited lighting is common in many larger offices. A few po-
sitions may be favoured but many will be in places where reflections on the screen are almost inevitable. Again some simple common sense precautions can be taken. A close-fitting cardboard
shield around the screen, painted black inside, is easy to make.

Poor ventilation and low humidity are also common features of
the multi-user office. Static electricity rises as humidity drops. All
computers and their peripherals give out heat and thus dry the
air. Static can be very harmful to any electronic apparatus and it is
not too good for human beings either, especially those with pace-
makers and similar devices. Some form of controlled 'draught' is
necessary as well as a means for keeping the temperature down
to a comfortable level. Better to work in a cool office and wear
enough clothes, than the other way round. The European Commission has issued a directive on this subject (number 90/270/
EC) which requires employers to evaluate the conditions under
which staff work and to supervise the taking of periodic rests.

Theft — your computer is at risk

Hardware theft Computer theft is increasing and the thieves are often well-in-
formed and selective, as the experience we report here shows.
Businesses with a high density of computer equipment which
provides the thief with plenty of choice are favoured targets. A
case was reported of thieves entering a large office where many
computers were installed. They switched each machine on, examined the programs on the hard disc and checked the RAM
available. If these fitted their 'shopping list', the machine was

taken. Organised, well planned and well informed operations of this kind are fuelled, it is suspected, by the opening up of new trade links with eastern Europe. Large offices are often easy to 'case'; strangers are not often questioned and 'workmen' wearing official-looking overalls are not even noticed. In this sort of situation it makes sense to purchase mid-range, less 'desirable' machines and to operate them via a file-server kept in a high security room. There are plenty of security programs available which prevent access to the hard disc and all its contents (see page 29). The RAM and programs cannot then be examined.

There are non-hardware thefts to consider also, particularly if **Software theft** you work in a multi-user situation, where others may have access to your machine. Not only is software commonly pirated but your 'original' material is also at risk. Again, a good security program is the answer. These are reviewed from time to time in computer magazines.

'Home' users such as small businesses, authors and illustrators should also take good care of their computer possessions for obviously these are now the major tools of their earning power. The loss of a machine can be serious but the loss of data even more devastating. What can we do to prevent disasters of this kind?

Sensible precautions

First. Do not advertise. Do not use your ground floor front room as an office, for every passer-by to see you at work with your highly desirable equipment. Convert the attic instead. If you have no alternative but the front room, then work out of view, perhaps behind a screen, and draw the curtains at night. Working behind a screen has the added advantage that it may help you to control unwanted reflection from the monitor screen.

Second. It is possible to purchase adhesive plates and a chain device which passes through rings on all the plates, being finally secured with a good quality padlock. The objective here is simply to make portable objects less portable.

Third. Make sure you have some kind of 'insurance-acceptable' locks to your house and to the windows, especially of the room where your equipment is. If you are settled in your house and not likely to move, then it is well worth considering laminated glass in the widows or as secondary glazing. This can be expensive but will probably not cost as much as special insurance premiums over a few years.

Fourth. If you are about to purchase a machine, consider the secondhand market. The thief is more likely to be looking for new, top-of-the-range models. If you have an old machine but

you want a 'faster' or 'better' one, consider upgrading your
present one, if it is possible to do so.

Fifth. Constantly save your work, i.e. every five minutes. Make a
backup at the end of every session, and make a third copy to keep
in another room. A whole book can use up quite a few floppy
discs and it is an advantage to use removable hard discs. Floppies
are great for the first back-up stage, but for long-term storage a
hard disc is often more convenient and less complicated. For example, a 44 megabyte removable hard disc is the equivalent of 40
to 50 floppies.

Other hazards

Virus infection Don't forget that the most destructive cause of data loss, and a
fairly common one, is a computer virus infection. There is no insurance here! Macintosh computers are less prone to infection,
and the anti-viral software is better than that available for MS-
DOS machines, but this can change at any time. Always use anti-
virus software. Never put in a 'foreign' disc without checking it
first. Be very cautious about networking. Use an isolated machine
if you use a modem. It is best to buy a cheap second-hand model
for receiving and sending messages. Never put this one on a network. Once a virus has entered a network community you are in
big trouble.

Dust All electronic devices are full of components that are electrostatic.
Computers have cooling slots and openings for discs, plugs etc.
This is where dust enters easily, attracted by all those electrically
charged bits and pieces. House and office cleaning make a cloud
of dust and dirt and a part of this tends to gradually build up in
unprotected machines. Always cover your computers, printers,
scanners, monitors etc. when not in use, but if a machine has been
left on all day then it makes sense to allow it to cool down for half
an hour first. Occasionally, suck the disc slots and other orifices
with a vacuum cleaner. This does not get at dirt deep inside the
machine but it does get at dirt near the disc heads. A professional
servicing is a good idea from time to time. How often this is necessary will depend on your local environment. Nearby building
works can create brick dust, a particularly dangerous ingredient
for computers.

Physical shock Never move a machine while it is switched on. The discs are spin-
ning at speeds in excess of 100 mph at their edges. The heads that
do the reading/writing to disc are floating above the disc surface
on a thin film of air. Thus air is both the lubricant and the cushion.
However, a sudden movement of the machine can exert powerful
centrifugal forces which are quite capable of seriously damaging
the heads and the hard disc and causing the destruction of data.

Most data storage is still on magnetised material. It is obvious *Magnetism*
therefore that items such as magnetic screwdrivers or telephones
with bells should be kept clear of computers. The increasing use
of optical storage devices will eliminate this particular risk.

It is advisable to protect all your computer equipment and related *Power sources*
devices with some form of power management system. Surges in
power supply when everybody switches on the electricity in the
evening can be enormous. The risks here vary with your location
and the time of day. Some countries have a particularly bad reputation in this respect, and a 'power cleaner' plug for computer users on the move is a good idea. Never switch computers on and
off in quick succession. They need time to discharge their electricity before coping with a new lot. An interval of ten seconds
should be allowed before restarting a machine.

Central heating, a nice dry atmosphere, nylon and wool clothes *Self-generated*
and a good soft pile carpet can generate thousands of volts in a *electricity*
few seconds and you are the unearthed battery that sends the
charge through your equipment. Quite enough to stop everything in its tracks. Some people are more 'generative' than others
but it is a very simple thing to remedy. An electricity-conducting
metal strip such as aluminium beading along the edge of your
work bench or desk, which is then wired to the central heating,
works very well. The beading needs to be placed where you just
can't help touching it, the less self-consciously the better. This
way you don't even have think about it. If the strip is placed correctly, you will touch it each time you use the keyboard. Anti-
electrostatic mats for placing under your keyboard, and larger
versions for placing under your chair, are available and these are
often advertised in computer journals.

Computers and printers also contribute to air drying. A relative *Humidity*
humidity of 65%–70% needs to be maintained for several reasons.
Your own personal working comfort is better at this sort of humidity level and there will be less likelihood of irritation to the
eyes through dryness. Paper for printing on also requires to be
kept at a reasonable level of humidity to prevent sheets sticking
together (static again). If you are in the habit of re-using 'waste'
sheets by turning them over for draft printing, remember the
point we made earlier. These sheets have not only been heated to
a high degree by the printer or photocopier but they have also re-
ceived negative and positive static charges. This is bound to make
them stick to each other unless they have been cooled and re-hu-
midified. The simplest form of humidifier is a water container attached to your radiator, but expensive custom-made equipment
is also available.

Keep in touch with user groups and read a journal relevant to *General advice*
your computer. New machines or methods of upgrading your old

one, and information concerning security, are common subjects. Lock up all your original program discs in another room and always keep your registration up to date. Although some software distributors offer to keep you posted, this is in fact a rarity. It saves money to upgrade your software each time a new version is published. There is often an offer for a free upgrade or an inexpensive one, but for a limited period. Once this time is up, you may have to pay the full price. A word of warning here. Following the 'don't advertise' rule, always post your registration cards in an envelope and not in their raw self-addressed state. This makes sure that your recently purchased expensive new program and its personal registration number are not going through the postal system on view to a large number of people.

Insurance

An institution with a building full of valuable equipment might choose to insure via a recognised insurance company. A lone author or illustrator may find that this may prove far too costly or feel that the risks are not so high as to be worth insurance cover. Why not, for instance, be your own insurance agent and simply build up an interest-earning fund to cover the purchase of a new or secondhand machine should yours get stolen or become unusable? Computer prices are falling steadily. Second-hand equipment, if privately owned, is likely to be in good condition and under-used. Lots of computer buffs are selling little-used machines because they have upgrade fever.

However, there are companies which specialise in computer insurance and we mention two here.

> **Tolson Messenger Ltd**
> Contact: The Commercial Manager, Mr Ian Jones
> *Telephone* 081 741 8361

> **National Vulcan Engineering Insurance Ltd**
> *Telephone* 061 834 8124

National Vulcan Insurance will not entertain an agreement unless you bolt down your computer equipment using special plates supplied by Intralink Associates Ltd and fixed on site by their engineers. All this costs money and fixes your equipment in one place. If you wish to move it to another location or even a different desk in the same room, you will not be able to do so without calling in Intralink. As a guide, the 1992 price for one fixing plate was about £60 plus VAT. Portable computers are a special problem. Vulcan may be able to offer insurance although there is a liability limit of £2500 on thefts from unattended vehicles.

Loss of data   Programs can always be re-installed but data loss is quite another matter since the data are very unlikely ever to be recovered. By far the most important aspect of data protection is the application of common sense: the regular back-up and duplication of material (see page 25). This is 100% up to you.

Consider your insurance position if you use your personal equipment at work as well as at home. Do not assume that because you have adequate cover for home use, it also extends to the office. If you borrow office equipment to use at home, will your employer cover the risk?

The multi-user situation

We have already mentioned the use of password-protected, file-serving arrangements for larger offices, but it is also advisable to have someone in authority who is responsible for the management of multi-user offices. This person should see that certain rules are applied. Loss of data in these situations is often caused by people leaving their work on machines which they intend to come back to later. In the meantime others may interfere with these files or bin them as junk. Individual users should never leave their work on a hard disc in a multi-user office but always transfer it back to a floppy of their own at the end of each session, taking care to remove any remaining material from the hard disc, thus leaving it 'clean' for other users. For everybody's sake, it is up to the manager to see that this happens.

Summary

Think about the room you work in: table-top space, the chair you sit on, lighting, and ventilation. Is the electricity supply adequate and is it properly earthed? Do you have *up-to-date* virus protection software running on your machine? Have you consulted an insurance company concerning your special needs? **Do you back-up your work often?** Do you keep spare copies of vital work at another location? If working in a multi-user office, make sure you do not leave your work on the hard disc when you finish a session, but always transfer it back again to your own floppy.

PUBLISHING AND THE LAW: COPYRIGHT AND AGREEMENTS

14

When you first discover the freedom and independence that desktop publishing gives, it's easy to forget that there are certain legal requirements that you must observe. UK and international law. Guidance for authors and illustrators who may need to sign agreements with publishers.

Publishing and the law

There is no way we can cover this subject in detail or replace the expertise of copyright lawyers. What we are keen to put across here is that you must be aware of some of the more general legal aspects of desktop authorship and publishing, so that you do not unwittingly contravene the law. As might be expected, 'ignorance is no defence'. We advise you to read the book mentioned under 'Further reading' for more detailed information.

What is 'publication'?

We note that there is a considerable degree of confusion about what constitutes publication. Cavendish and Pool, in their book on copyright, spend a few pages on the various meanings of the term. We are going to take one of the easier definitions, one that applies in many cases to scientific work.

'Publication' is when a work is made in multiple copies and is offered to the public. It does not have to be for sale, it merely has to be 'offered'. For those engaged in teaching this may have legal implications if copyright material is included in lecture notes or handouts 'offered' to others.

Copyright

All literary and artistic work, *in whatever form,* is copyright. 'In whatever form' means exactly what it says: it might be invisibly electronic or a physically tangible piece of paper. Although an author's, artist's or photographer's copyright may cease fifty years (70 years from 1995) after the year of his or her death, there is usually copyright attached to the printed or published item itself. For example, Homer's 'Iliad' may no longer be the copyright of Homer himself but the book, the translation, the typography and the design may each separately or together be the copyright of the translator, publisher or printer, and these rights may still be extant. Thus copyright exists not only in the text and illustrations being presented, but also in the *form* of their presentation. Basically there is no copyright in ideas while they reside only in your mind, but the minute you express them they become your 'intellectual property'. You are, of course, on rather shaky ground if you are called upon to prove this and it can be important to record ideas in some form. Before 1988 it was possible for a person to make a recording of an extempore speech and then print it claiming the copyright of the speech, since it was now in recorded form. Since the new Copyright Act of 1988 (in force since 1st August 1989) this is no longer possible. Whoever records a speech, the copyright in it belongs to the speaker. It may be desirable to have evidence of the date on which the speech was made. This may be done by keeping a copy of dated program notes and it is particularly easy to establish the date of creation when computers are used for notes or any other document, since this date and dates of amendment are automatically recorded as part of the file.

Employment If you are employed under a 'contract of service' the copyright of your work belongs to your employer. Consider the effect of this within a university. It has been common practice for the head of a research group to assume that work done under his/her authority belongs to the person who did it, and this assumed ownership can extend to others whose job it is to provide associated services, such as artists and photographers. This is not the case. The employer has all the rights, unless formal written agreements have been made to the contrary. If your contract is part-time you may need to establish exactly what your employer expects to own. A 'contract of service' is not the same as a 'contract for services'. The latter is usually a specific agreement for a particular piece of work, the copyright remaining with the creator unless otherwise agreed. Copyright is a 'negative' right. It gives the owner power to *prevent* publication, it does not confer the right to publish.

Multi-ownership Copyright might be owned by more than one person as in multi-authored work, and as this may present difficulties later it may be reasonable for the publisher of the work to seek assignment of copyright from the contributors. Photography has often been the subject of contention in the past. There are many situations in commercial photography where it may not be clear who the photographer is. Prior to 1989 it was the commissioner of the photograph, or if it was not commissioned, the owner of the film upon which the first image was recorded, who had the copyright in it. This is no longer the case. The first copyright holder in any photographic image is the 'person responsible for the making of the photograph'. This is not necessarily the person pressing the button or any other person associated only with the photographic technicalities of production.

Prior to the 1988 Act, the commissioner of any photograph or a painted or drawn portrait owned the copyright in it. This is no longer the case. The act of commissioning any work does not automatically confer copyright ownership on the commissioner. In science, a person may commission an artist to illustrate an idea formed in the commissioner's mind. The commissioner can always lay claim to the idea, but the visual creation of that idea on paper, film, tape or any electronic medium is someone else's work and the copyright belongs to the creator. This does not, however, apply to typists who wordprocess from dictation or a draft document. This is because their work is not regarded as creative. **Commissioning**

Purchasing a 'work' does not confer copyright ownership on the purchaser. If you want to own the copyright in any work you have not produced yourself you have to negotiate for it. **Purchase of work**

Authors, artists and photographers, particularly those who work on a freelance basis, need to consider the above points with care. Your copyright is also your bread and butter and it is inadvisable to relinquish it carelessly or by default. There are many ways in which copyright can be retained while still allowing a third party, a publisher for example, to use your work to your mutual advantage.

The major alternative is to grant a 'licence for use'. This can take many forms. A licence can be exclusive or non-exclusive, limited to time, to geographic location, to one particular mode of reproduction but not another, or any combination of these. The copyright itself can also be granted for a limited period and then recalled. It may be in your interest to grant copyright to a publisher only while a publication remains in print, for example. **Licensing**

Apart from the UK, copyright law applies to all countries who have signed the Berne Convention and/or the Universal Copyright Convention. More than one hundred countries have now agreed to abide by international copyright law. These countries are referred to in the Copyright Act as 'acceptable countries' and they recognise each other's laws. **International conventions**

To gain at least the minimum protection at international level, you must use the © symbol and state the year, author, publisher and country of origin, on your publication.

Qualifying persons A person cannot claim copyright under UK law unless he or she is a 'qualifying person'. This means a person who is a national of an 'acceptable country' or domiciled in the UK.

Duration The duration of copyright in literary or artistic work normally runs for fifty years starting from the end of the year in which the author of a work dies (from July 1st 1995 it will be life plus 70 years). In the case of multi-authored work, copyright runs from the end of the year in which the remaining living author dies.

Registration Do not be deceived into thinking that the Copyright Receipt Office can provide you with some form of copyright registration. This Office does not accept unpublished manuscripts or typescripts. Registration of material in order to prove copyright ownership at a later date ceased in 1842. Now all work, whether published or not, is copyright once it has been put into a form that can eventually be visually perceived, including via an electronic retrieval system. However, if it seems really vital to establish your claim to authorship, it is still possible to register material by depositing it at the following address:

> **The Stationers' Company**
> Stationers' Hall
> Ave Maria Lane
> London EC4M 7DD
> *Telephone* 071 248 2934

As far as computer origination of material is concerned, either the hardcopy printout or the electronic version on disc can be deposited and recorded. You can also deposit a copy of your material with your solicitor or bank, making sure, of course, that it is dated.

Agreements

These are not necessarily complex legal documents, but can be simply written letters between the interested parties stating what each wants and expects from the other. We say 'written' because some form of hardcopy is essential in case of litigation later. An agreement should cover the following: ownership of the work; ownership of the copyright; payment of fees, the amount and when; what rights are being granted; arbitration procedures and a termination clause. Beware of signing an agreement that may involve other people. It is very common for authors to find that they have signed an agreement to supply illustrative material as well as text. This is often a recipe for serious financial cost to the author. In book publishing agreements, try to make sure that the publisher agrees to publish by a certain date, so that if this does not occur the agreement is void and you will be able to regain all your rights as well as your material.

Copyright, licensing and the fine points of signing agreements are all minefields for the unwary. Whenever very important issues have to be faced, it is worth seeking an expert opinion and/or the advice of your professional society if you have one. We can thoroughly recommend all authors as well as illustrators closely involved in publication to join the Society of Authors, who have considerable experience in dealing with agreements.

Society of Authors
84 Drayton Gardens
London SW 10 9SB
Telephone 071 373 6642 Fax 071 373 5768

Copying

The most usual form of copying is via the photocopier. The 1988 Copyright Act still retains the former Act's permission to allow copying in limited amounts for private study and research, or for the purpose of writing a criticism or review. Most public libraries now have strict rules concerning copying and the person wanting to copy may have to sign an undertaking that the copying is for private use only. There may also be a licence fee.

What you **MAY NOT** do:

- Make use of any copyright material without the permission of the copyright holder and previously published source.

- Make multiple copies, or copies for other people.

- Offer copyrighted work for sale, e.g. as part of lecture notes.

What you **MAY** do:

- Copy a document for your own *private* study and research (i.e. not for incorporation into lecture notes or to be displayed as a slide or OHP transparency). If the copying is done at a centre *registered for the purpose* (most university libraries, for example, fall into this category), you may be asked to sign a declaration that you will abide by the law.

- Copy a limited amount for the purposes of criticism or review. The law states that the amount copied for this purpose should not be a 'substantial part' of the document in question, but it does not define how much is a 'substantial part'. Our advice is to use common sense and only use a 'small part' for review purposes.

For further information contact:

The Patent Office
Industrial Property & Copyright Department
Copyright Enquiries
45 Southampton Buildings
London WC2A 1AR
Telephone 071 438 4700

The British Copyright Council
Copyright House
29-33 Berners Street
London WC1R 4TP
Telephone 071 829 6145 x 8342

Collecting Societies

These societies act as agents for the collection of fees due to members from the use of their work. Authors and artists may not always be aware that copying of their work is being done or that use is being made of it by others. An extract from a book used in a radio or TV broadcast, or an illustration for a textbook that appears in a sales brochure without authorisation, are examples of this. These societies are affiliated to other similar international organisations, so that monitoring may be very extensive.

The Authors' Licensing and Collecting Society
33-34 Alfred Place
London WC1E 7DP
Telephone 071 255 2034 *Fax* 071 323 0486

Design and Artists' Copyright Society
St Mary's Clergy House
Whitechurch Lane
London E1 7QR
Telephone 071 247 1650 *Fax* 071 377 5855

Legal deposit in the British Library

The law relating to legal deposit is really part of the Copyright Act. Compliance with the Act is usually the publisher's responsibility not the author's.

Further information is obtainable from:

The British Library
Legal Deposit Office
Boston Spa
Wetherby, Yorkshire
Telephone 0937 546268

International Standard Book Numbers

All published works in the form of books are required to have a unique ISBN number. Apply to the following address:

Standard Book Numbering Agency
12 Dyot Street
London WC1A 1DE
Telephone 071 836 8911

Data Protection Act

This is a law that requires all users of computers to register if they have *any kind* of personal data held in an electronic file. This means that if you hold even an address book in digital form you have to register. You can have a handwritten address book at home with all kinds of highly personal things in it, but you can't hold any sort of personal details about other people in digital form without registration. Failure to register under this Act is against the law in the UK and is subject to substantial fines. The law came into force on 11th November 1987.

For details concerning application forms, and to find out if the law applies to you, contact:

Data Protection Registrar
Springfield House
Water Lane
Wilmslow
Cheshire SK9 5AX
Telephone 0625 535777 or 535711

Summary

Seek expert advice, especially when other persons are involved in your work. It is always advisable to try and retain your copyright where possible and particularly so in important work such as book publication. Multi-author work may be an exception to this. Joining a professional society, such as the Society of Authors or one of the Collecting Societies may be very helpful when you need expert advice.

GLOSSARY

Words in italics are separately defined.

A

alphabet length The space occupied by the 26 *lowercase letters* in a given *typeface* and size, when they are set in a single line without spaces.

alphanumerics Letters and numbers, as opposed to other kinds of symbol.

application (Macintosh) Any program that is designed to manipulate data in a particular way. For example, 'write' and 'draw' programs are applications, but systems programs are not.

artwork Text or *graphics* presented in a form suitable for reproduction. In desktop publishing, the artwork is usually in the form of output from a *laserprinter*.

ascender The part of a *lowercase letter*, such as 'd' or 'h', that rises above the *x-height*.

ASCII American Standard Code for Information Interchange. A system of codes used to represent the *character* set in a computer.

ASPIC A *generic coding* system recommended by the British Printing Industries Federation.

asymmetric layout A page layout that has no central axis. Typically, both headings and text would be *ranged left*.

B

back-edge In a bound document, the edge of the page nearest to the binding.

baseline An imaginary horizontal line on which the bases of most *lowercase letters* (i.e. those without *descenders*) are aligned.

baseline-to-baseline measurement The measurement (usually in *points*) from the baseline of one line of type to the baseline of the next. *See also*: linefeed.

binary The counting system used in computing. The binary system uses the base 2, as opposed to the decimal system which uses the base 10.

bit Stands for 'binary information transfer'. The bit is the basic unit of information in computer systems. Each bit can have a value of either 0 or 1.

bitmapping The storage of an image in terms of *pixels* and their specific locations.

body size The term originates from metal type and it refers to the size of the 'body' on which each *character* is cast. The body size, usually measured in *points*, is the vertical dimension of the surfaces carrying the characters. With *digital type* there is no physical body, so the term has little relevance. *See also*: point size.

boot-up Computer slang for switching your computer on.

brightness The perceived attribute of a colour that allows it to be classed on a scale ranging from very dim (or dark) to very bright. Brightness is the perception associated with the *luminance* of a surface and is therefore a property of both the object itself and the amount of light illuminating it. On VDUs, changes in luminance will cause changes in both *lightness* and brightness.

byte A measure of computer storage. A byte is equal to one character in an eight-bit environment.

C

cap. height *See*: capital letter height.

capital letter height The height of the capital letters in a given *typeface* and size, measured from the *baseline* to the *capital line*.

capital line An imaginary line running along the tops of the capital letters in a line of type set in a given *typeface* and size.

caption Text explaining an illustration. Not to be confused with a legend or key.

central processing unit (often abbreviated to CPU) The part of the computer that sorts data and executes commands from the programs or the keyboard.

centred setting The setting of text such that

each line is filled to the nearest whole word, with word and letter spacing held constant; the line is then centred between the lefthand and righthand margins.

character A letter, numeral, punctuation mark, other symbol or space.

character-driven A computer system with fixed character shapes stored in the *ROM*. Data manipulation and display are controlled by typing commands at the keyboard. *See also*: graphics-driven.

chromatic aberration Blurring and depth effects in coloured images, caused by the fact that different wavelengths of light are bent by different amounts as they enter the eye.

clipboard The place where information that has been cut or copied is held, until such time as another item is cut or copied.

CISC Complex Instruction Set Computing. A standard for microprocessor chips used in computers. Has reached the limits of development and is being superceeded by the more efficient *RISC* standard.

CMYK A system used for specifying the amounts of the *process colours* needed to reproduce an artwork colour in print. The process colours are *cyan, magenta* and yellow plus black.

colour separation The process of photographing or electronically scanning a coloured image to produce four separate images representing the red, green, blue and black components of the original. In printing, the four images are superimposed to recreate the original colours. The ink colours used are black and the *process colours. See also*: four-colour printing.

command-driven Used to describe a computer system where the user must type commands at the keyboard. *See also*: menu-driven.

complementary colour The complementary of a colour is produced when that colour is removed from white light. If blue is removed, the remaining wavelengths are mainly red and green, giving yellow as the complementary colour. Thus the complementary of a *primary colour* of light is in effect a mixture of the two remaining primaries.

continuous tone Used to describe an image that contains a range of tonal values, such as a photograph. *See also*: halftone.

copyfitting Calculating how many lines your copy will occupy when set in a given *typeface* and type size, and to a given line length.

counter An enclosed or partially enclosed space within a character.

CPU *See*: central processing unit.

crop marks *See*: trim marks.

cursor A moveable indicator on the screen, used to select the point in the data at which the next command is to be actioned.

cut-and-paste Editing operations that allow the removal of portions of text from a document and their reinstatement elsewhere in the same document or in another document.

cyan A mixture of blue and green, one of the three *process colours* in printing.

D

daisywheel printer A printing device with the character forms held on a metal disc.

data Information (always plural).

descender The part of a *lowercase letter*, such as 'g' or 'y', that drops below the *baseline*.

desk accessories (Macintosh) Mini-applications that are available whilst you are using any other application. Examples include the Calculator, Alarm Clock and *Scrapbook*.

desktop The working area on the screen. Also the highest (first) level in the *hierarchical filing system*.

device independence *See*: output-device independence.

diazo A contact printing process in which ammonia is used as the developing agent in an ultraviolet light source. Commonly used to produce slides with white lettering on a blue ground. The process is unstable and slides are apt to fade.

digital type Type that is held only in electronic form.

dingbats A font consisting of non-*alphanumeric* typographic elements (symbols) of various kinds.

disc drive A mechanism for holding a disc, and for writing information on it and retrieving information from it.

display sizes Type sizes of 18 *points* and upwards.

document (Macintosh) The name given to a file created within an *application*.

dominant wavelength The wavelength of light most heavily represented in a colour.

dot-matrix printer A printing device on which the characters are formed by different configurations of pins striking the paper. There are normally either nine or twenty-four pins.

double-page spread A pair of facing pages. Two A4 pages will of course give an A3 spread.

dpi Abbreviation for 'dots per inch'.

draft-quality output Many dot-matrix printers offer two or more printing qualities. Draft output is usually the fastest and lowest quality option. *See also*: letter-quality output, near-letter-quality output.

drag and drop Replaces cut and paste in some programs, allowing you to select an object and drag it to a new location. In some illustration programs it will allow you to drag colours from a swatch to fill an area, for example. Saves time. *See also* OLE.

driver A computer *program* or device that communicates with a *peripheral* device such as a printer or disc drive.

drop cap. Short for 'drop capital'. Often used at the beginning of a chapter or paragraph, this is a capital letter that extends below the *baseline* of the first line of type, and perhaps several subsequent lines.

dry-transfer lettering Lettering attached to a carrier sheet is transferred to the *artwork* by rubbing the back of the carrier. Letraset is the best-known brand. Dry-transfer lettering is expensive to buy and requires a certain amount of skill for good results. Computer graphics has largely replaced this method of lettering.

dummy A model or mock-up of a document, used as a guide for pagination, imposition, folding and binding.

E

electronic typesetting Methods of typesetting in which the type is held in electronic (i.e. digital) form.

em The width of a *lowercase* letter 'm'. This is usually the same as the *point size* of the type. Thus an em in 10pt type will be 10 points wide. The em is used as a unit of measurement for horizontal space on a line. Indents, for example, are usually specified in ems. *See also*: pica em.

en The width of a *lowercase* 'n'. This is usually half the width of the *em*, i.e. half the *point size* of the type in question. Ens are used to specify small amounts of horizontal space, for example between an index entry and its associated page number.

F

file A collection of information stored on a disc. Each *document, application, desk accessory* etc. constitutes a file.

fill pattern Patterns and shadings used to fill objects in 'paint' and 'draw' programs.

filmsetting *See*: phototypesetting.

finder (Macintosh) Program responsible for retrieving files when you ask for them.

floppy disc Flexible plastic disc used for the magnetic storage of information. The most commonly used sizes are 3.5in and 5.25in.

fixed space A unit of horizontal space, such as an *em* or an *en*, that remains unchanged during *justification* and *hyphenation*.

flush-left setting The setting of text such that all lines begin at the lefthand margin but do not necessarily end exactly at the righthand margin. Each line is filled to the nearest whole word, with *word spacing* and *letter spacing* held constant. *Hyphenation* is usually confined to exceptionally long words. *See also*: flush-right setting.

flush-right setting The setting of text such that all lines end exactly at the righthand margin, but do not necessarily begin exactly at the lefthand margin. As with *flush-left setting*, each line is filled to the nearest whole word, with *word spacing* and *letter spacing* held constant, and *hyphenation* is usually confined to exceptionally long words. *See also*: flush-left setting.

folder *Documents* and *applications* can be grouped inside folders on the *desktop*. This reduces clutter and makes it easier to find your *files*. Folders can in turn be placed in other folders. This is called the *hierarchical filing system*.

folio Page number.

font Traditionally, a font is a set of letters, numerals, punctuation marks and other *characters* in the same *typeface, type style* and size. With metal type, the printer holds a separate font, or set of characters, for every combination of size and style likely to be needed in a given typeface. With *digital type*, however, a number of sizes and styles can be generated from the same 'font master' held in electronic form. In the computer world, the word 'font' is increasingly used to mean 'typeface' rather than a specific combination of typeface, style and size. *See also*: printer fonts; screen fonts.

fore-edge In a document, the edge of the page farthest from the binding.

fount An alternative spelling for *font*.

four-colour printing Four *colour separations* are screen-printed on top of one another using the three *process colours* and black. Dots of different sizes and colours combine to recreate the colours of the original. *See also*: screen printing.

G

galley proof A proof in which the text is not divided into pages. *See also*: page proof.

generic coding The insertion of codes into electronic text to identify structural elements such as paragraphs, listed points, headings at various levels, and so on. The codes are later converted to typesetting instructions. This procedure allows output from relatively unsophisticated wordprocessing systems to be used for *electronic typesetting*. It is not necessary with '*WYSIWYG*' systems such as the Apple Macintosh. In the computer environment, generic codes are control codes for the program.

global search and replace *See*: search and replace.

graphic design Designing with type and 'pictures'. *See also*: graphics.

graphics A loosely-used term, generally taken to mean illustrations or 'pictures' as opposed to text. A graphic may include lines, shadings, alphanumerics and other symbols. In computing, however, the term is used specifically to mean the images created by a *graphics-driven* computer where every *pixel* is directly addressable by the *software*.

graphics-driven A computer system where the character shapes are not fixed in the *ROM*. Shapes, including characters, can be created using menus and a pointing device. *See also*: character-driven.

grey scale The range of tones between black and white.

grid The grid defines the margins and text area on a page. The text area itself may be divided into two, three, four or more columns into which all text and illustrations must fit exactly.

gutter The space between columns of text. Sometimes *back-edge* margins are referred to as 'gutter margins'.

H

h & j Short for 'hyphenation and justification'. H & j routines are computer programs used to achieve a straight, or 'justified', righthand margin. *See also*: hyphenation, justified setting.

hairline rule A rule that is 0.25 of a point in width.

halftone A method of reproducing a *continuous tone* image such as a photograph. The image is photographed through a screen. Lighter areas are reproduced as smaller dots farther apart, while darker areas consist of larger dots closer together. *See also*: screen printing.

hanging indent Where the first line of a paragraph is against the lefthand margin and subsequent lines in the paragraph are indented.

hard disc A disc that is permanently encased in the *disk drive*. Hard discs (sometimes referred to as 'Winchesters') have a much greater storage capacity and speed than *floppy discs*.

hardcopy Printout from a computer *file*. Written or typed copy may also be referred to as hardcopy.

hardware The equipment, as opposed to the *software*, comprising a computer system.

hierarchical filing system A filing system where files can be placed inside folders, which in turn can be placed inside other folders, and so on.

HLS A system of specifying colours according to *hue* (expressed as an angle), *light-*

ness (expressed as a percentage) and *saturation* (also expressed as a percentage).

hot-link Data can be hot-linked to the chart derived from them, so that changes in data will be automatically reflected in the chart. Very useful when updating work. Hot-linking is being increasingly used in a variety of applications. *See also:* OLE.

house style A set of rules relating to typography and to linguistic matters such as spelling, abbreviation and punctuation. Normally all publications from the same publisher or company would be expected to conform to these rules.

hue That property of a colour which is determined by its dominant wavelength.

hyphenation The breaking of words at ends of lines in *justified setting*. A good hyphenation routine breaks words only at legitimate points.

I

I-beam A type of *cursor* frequently used in text-handling programs.

icon A small picture used to represent an object (such as a *file*), a concept or a message.

illuminance A measure of the amount of light falling on a surface, or on the eye when looking directly at a light source.

imagesetter A *laser typesetter*.

impact printer A printing device in which the paper is struck by a character form (*daisywheel printers*) or a configuration of pins (*dotmatrix printers*).

imposition The arrangement of a number of pages of camera-ready copy so that they can be printed together on one sheet of paper. The arrangement must be such that the pages will be in the correct sequence when the sheet is folded and trimmed.

initialise Before a disc can be used to store data, it must be initialised. The available storage space is divided into segments so that the system can keep a record of what has been stored where on the disc.

inkjet printer A printing device on which characters are formed by tiny jets of ink squirted at the paper in a dot matrix configuration.

install Some programs cannot be used immediately simply by inserting the *floppy*

disc into the computer. Such programs need to be installed. This is often a matter of selecting the parts of the program that are appropriate for your system, so that in effect you have a customised version of the program.

intensity *See*: tonal value.

interface The link between two parts of a computer system, or between the computer system and the operator (human/computer interface).

J

justification *See*: justified setting.

justified setting The setting of text so that all lines are of exactly the same length, thus creating a straight righthand margin as well as a straight lefthand margin. This is achieved by hyphenating words at ends of lines where necessary, and by varying word spacing and letter spacing. *See also*: hyphenation.

K

kerning The adjustment of spacing between individual pairs of letters so that the letters in a word appear evenly spaced. In automatic kerning systems, each letter pair is looked up in a table and the spacing adjusted according to the value specified. This requires a considerable amount of memory, so many systems offer manual kerning only. Here the operator can move individual letters at will. This facility is especially useful for words set in capital letters and in *display sizes*. *See also*: letterspacing, tracking.

key synonymous with legend. Text and/or symbols explaing a diagram, chart or graph and often incorporated within the artwork area

kilobyte (often abbreviated to K) 1024 *bytes*, or about 1000 characters.

L

label Text identifying parts of an illustration, or other texts.

LAN *See*: local area network.

landscape format A page format in which the horizontal dimension is the longest.

lasercopier A high-quality xerographic copier using laser technology. Not to be confused with *laserprinters*. *See also*: xerography.

laserprinter A printing device which uses

xerography and laser technology. Laser-printers are capable of generating traditional printers' typefaces at resolutions of around 300dpi. New models, now on sale, print at resolutions of 400 to 600dpi.

lasersetter *See*: laser typesetter.

laser typesetter A typesetting machine based on laser technology. Laser typesetters produce graphic arts quality output at resolutions of 1280dpi and above.

leader dots Rows of dots used to guide the eye across the page, typically between columns of information.

leader lines Hairline rules used to lead the eye from a label outside a drawing to a point within a drawing.

leading Space added between lines of type (usually specified in *points*). The term originates from metal type, where thin strips of lead can be inserted between lines, but it has no real meaning when applied to digital type and is best avoided. Some page make-up programs refer to 'leading' when they mean *line spacing* or *linefeed*.

legend see key.

letter-quality output (often abbreviated to LQ) The highest quality of output obtainable from an *impact printer*. Only *daisywheel printers* are capable of true letter-quality. *See also*: draft-quality output, near-letter-quality output.

letter spacing The space between letters making up a word. *See also*: kerning, letterspacing, tracking.

letterspacing The addition of space between letters. Letterspacing is sometimes used in headings, supposedly to give them more impact. It may also occur in *justified setting* if adjustments to the inter-word spacing alone would result in too much white space on a line. *See also*: kerning, tracking.

lightness The perceived attribute of a colour which allows it to be classed on a scale ranging from very dark to very light. Lightness is the perception associated with the *reflectance* of a surface, and it is therefore a property of the surface itself.

line increment *See*: linefeed.

line spacing The space between lines of type, measured from the *baseline* of one line of text to the baseline of the next

(usually specified in *points*, sometimes in millimetres). *See also*: linefeed.

linefeed The distance between the *baseline* of one line of type and the baseline of the next. Linefeed is usually measured in *points*, but in some circumstances it may be more convenient to use millimetres. (With metal type, the linefeed is equal to the *body size* of the type plus any *leading*. Thus, 10pt type with two points of leading would have a 12pt linefeed.)

lining numerals Numerals that are aligned top and bottom with the *baseline* and *capital line*, as opposed to *non-lining numerals* with *ascenders* and *descenders*. Also known as 'modern' numerals.

litho *See*: offset lithography.

local area network A group of *microcomputers* and *peripherals* with direct (i.e. cable) links between them, operating within a limited geographical area (for example, in the same building or the same room).

lock In most systems, individual *documents* or whole discs can be locked to prevent them from being edited, renamed, or accidentally erased.

lowercase letters Small letters, as opposed to capital or *uppercase* letters. So called because of the position of the wooden 'cases' in which metal type is traditionally kept.

LQ *See*: letter-quality output.

luminance A measure of the intensity of light reflected or emitted from a surface. It depends on both *illuminance* and *reflectance* and takes into account the fact that the sensitivity of the eye is not the same for all wavelengths of light. The perception of *brightness* is approximately correlated with luminance.

M

magenta A mixture of blue and red, one of the *process colours* in printing.

MB *See*: megabyte.

mean line An imaginary line running along the top of the *lowercase* letters in a line of type set in a given face and size.

measure The width of the column in which lines of type are set, i.e. the line length. The measure may be specified in *picas*, inches or metric units.

mechanical tint Patterns or shading used to fill areas in *graphics*. Obtainable in 'paint' and 'draw' programs, and in the form of *dry-transfer* sheets.

megabyte   (often abbreviated to MB) 1,024,000 *bytes*, or about 1 million characters.

menu   A list of possible actions, displayed on the screen.

menu-driven   A computer system which the user operates by selecting alternatives from a menu. Selection may be by means of a pointing device (such as a *mouse*), or by typing very simple commands (such as a letter or numeral plus the return key). *See also*: command-driven.

microcomputer   A small computer. The term is derived from the 'micro' chip used to construct the processor.

modern numerals   *See*: lining numerals.

modem   A device that enables a computer to communicate with another computer via the telephone net work.

monitor   A *VDU* that shows what the computer is doing.

monochrome   Usually used to refer to black-and-white images, but any image with lettering or graphics in a single colour on a black or white background is a form of monochrome image.

monoline   Used to describe typefaces in which the strokes forming the letters have a constant, or nearly constant, width.

monospaced characters   Characters that occupy the same amount of horizontal space on the line, regardless of their width. They are a hangover from the mechanical typewriter and are typical of the less expensive kinds of impact printer. *See also*: proportional spacing.

mouse   A pointing device used with *menu-driven* and *graphics-driven* systems. The movement of the mouse on a flat surface controls the movement of the *cursor* on the screen.

MS-DOS   The Microsoft Disc Operating System, used by the IBM-PC and compatible computers.

multi-tasking   Multi-tasking systems are able to perform several tasks at the same time. For example, the user may be able to edit one document while printing another.

multi-user   Describes a computer system that allows several users to access the same machine, programs and data files at the same time.

N

near-letter-quality output   This is the highest quality of output that most dotmatrix printers can achieve. It is relatively slow. *See also*: draft-quality output, letter-quality output.

network   *See*: local area network.

NLQ   *See*: near-letter-quality output.

non-lining numerals   Numerals with *ascenders* and *descenders* (also known as 'old-style' numerals).

O

offset lithography   A printing process that is much used for output from desktop-publishing systems. The finished pages are photographed to create film negatives, and these in turn are used to create printing plates. Ink adheres to the image areas and is repelled by non-image areas. The plate is attached to a cylinder, and the ink is transferred to the paper via an intermediate cylinder.

old-style numerals   *See*: non-lining numerals.

OLE   Object Linking and Embedding. Some programs allow you to 'cut and paste' or '*drag and drop*' objects between each other. These objects can remain linked to the originating program, so that changes made at the point of origin are automatically transferred to the destination document.

opacity   A characteristic of paper. The greater the opacity, the less *show-through* there will be. Heavier papers are not necessarily more opaque than lighter ones.

operating system   A program that organises the activities of the computer and its *peripheral* devices.

orphan   The first line of a paragraph, isolated at the bottom of a column or page.

outline-mapping   The storage of an image in terms of outlines with no fixed dimensions.

output-device independence   A facility provided by certain programming languages used for specifying output. The contents of pages are described in such a way that they can be output on any compatible device. *See also*: page-description language.

P

package Program or programs bought 'off-the-shelf', as opposed to being written for a specific purpose.

page-description language A computer-programming language used to control output. The language is used to describe the nature of the text and graphic elements on a page, and their exact placement. Any output device that is capable of supporting a specific page-description language can accept pages from any program that is capable of generating pages in that language. The pages are thus held in a form that is *output-device independent*.

page grid *See*: grid.

page proof A proof in which the text and any illustrations have been made up into pages. Page proofs show the final appearance of each page. *See also*: galley proof.

Pantone™ (USA) The first scientific colour specification system for defining printers' *CMYK* colours. There are now several such systems in use.

parameter A variable that can be set at a particular value to suit a specific operation.

parentheses Round brackets (as opposed to square brackets).

pass One run through a computer system.

PC *See*: personal computer.

peripheral An input or output device that is separate from the computer itself, e.g. a scanner or a laserprinter.

personal computer (often abbreviated to PC) *See*: microcomputer.

photocopying A relatively cheap and readily available method of producing a few copies of a document. *Xerography* is the most commonly used process.

photomechanical transfer (often abbreviated to PMT) A method of making high-quality photographic copies of *artwork*. The image is exposed onto light-sensitive paper to give a negative. A positive is then made by a contact printing process involving the chemical transfer of the image onto a second sheet of paper.

phototypesetting A method of typesetting in which the characters are exposed onto photographic paper or film. The characters may be held in the form of a physical matrix of some kind, or they may be held in digital form. Digital characters may be 'painted' onto a CRT (cathode ray tube) which is then exposed onto the photographic material, or they may be written directly onto the photographic material by a laser (*laser typesetting*).

pi font A set of special characters such as mathematical symbols.

pica A pica is equal to 12 *points*, or approximately one sixth of an inch.

pica em A pica em is a 12pt *em*, i.e. the width of a *lowercase* 'm' in a 12pt type size. The pica em is a unit of horizontal spacing and it can be used with type of any size. When dealing with ems, it is important to be sure whether they are pica ems, or whether they relate to the size of type being set.

picture element *See*: pixel.

pitch The number of *monospaced characters* per horizontal inch. Used as a measure of character size. Impact printers may offer 10 pitch, 12 pitch, 15 pitch and 17 pitch, but 10 and 12 pitch are the most common.

pixel The smallest element that can be displayed on a computer screen. On a colour display, each pixel consists of three differently coloured phosphor dots.

platemaking The process of making printing plates for *offset lithography* by photographing *artwork*.

plotter A *peripheral* device capable of receiving instructions from a computer and drawing graphics at very high resolution according to those instructions. These machines 'draw' in increments as small as 0.005in (0.1mm).

PMT *See*: photomechanical transfer.

point (often abbreviated to 'pt') A point is approximately equal to 1/72 of an inch (or 0.013837 of an inch, to be precise). The point is the basic unit in the system of measurement traditionally used by printers.

point size The traditional way of specifying type sizes. The system originates from metal type, where each character is cast on a metal body. The measurement in *points* relates to the vertical dimension of the surfaces carrying the characters. As the point size is not a direct measurement of the characters themselves, the apparent size of characters of the same point size varies from one *typeface* to another. Even though *digital type* has no physical 'body', the same system of measurement is still widely used. For some purposes, however, it is more convenient to measure the capital-letter height or the x-height of the type in millimetres.

port A socket on a computer, into which a *peripheral* device can be plugged.

portrait format A page format in which the vertical dimension is the longest.

PostScript A proprietary *page-description language* marketed by Adobe Systems. It is currently the most popular of such languages and has been adopted by both Apple and IBM as a standard.

primary colour One of a set of three colours from which most other colours can be mixed. When coloured lights are mixed, the primaries are red, blue and green; when pigments are mixed the primaries are a bluish red (*magenta*), a bluish green (*cyan*), and yellow. *See also:* complementary colour.

print buffer A block of *random-access memory* set aside to provide temporary storage for files that are waiting to be printed.

printer fonts Fonts used by *laserprinters* and *laser typesetters. See also:* screen fonts.

printer resolution The number of dots per inch that a printer or typesetter is capable of generating. Resolution varies from perhaps 72dpi on an *impact printer* to 300-600dpi on a *laserprinter* and over 2000dpi on some *laser typesetters.*

process camera A camera specifically designed for the various photographic processes involved in printing.

process colours In printing, all colours can be reproduced by combinations of the three process colours, yellow, *cyan* and *magenta*, plus black. Each colour is printed from a separate plate.

program A set of instructions that enables a computer to carry out a particular operation or series of operations.

proportional spacing A system of spacing whereby the amount of space each character occupies on a line depends on the width of that character. Some *impact printers* offer a form of proportional spacing, but satisfactory proportional spacing can be achieved only with printers' *typefaces* and a *laserprinter* or *laser typesetter. See also:* monospaced characters.

pt Abbreviation for *'point'.*

publication 'A work is said to be published when copies of it are issued to the public. The place of publication, the nature of the imprint and the size of distribution are immaterial...'. (Quoted from: Legal Deposits in the British Library.)

pull-down menu A *menu* whose presence is indicated only by its title. The options are revealed when the title is activated in some way, usually by pointing at it with a device such as a *mouse*. Once an option has been selected, the menu disappears again, leaving the screen uncluttered.

R

ragged-left setting *See*: flush-right setting.

ragged-right setting *See*: flush-left setting.

RAM *See*: random-access memory.

random-access memory The part of the computer's *resident memory* that is used for the temporary storage of programs and data files currently in use. It can be both written to and read from. It is erased when the power is switched off.

ranged-left setting *See*: flush-left setting.

ranged-right setting *See*: flush-right setting.

raster image processor (often abbreviated to RIP) A device that receives data from a computer and uses *PostScript* for typesetting.

read-only memory (ROM) The part of the computer's resident memory that is used for storing *programs, fonts,* and other essential data needed by the computer and the printer. It is not erased when the power is switched off.

reflectance The percentage of incident light which is reflected from a surface. Reflectance is perceived as *lightness.*

refresh rate Images on a *VDU* are created by electrons hitting the phosphor coating of the screen and causing it to glow. It is not necessary for the image to glow continuously for it to be perceived as steady, so it is typically refreshed at a rate of 50 times per second with European voltage systems and at 60 times per second on American systems. The higher the refresh rate, the less the perceptible flicker in the image.

register marks These are crossed hairlines placed outside the print area and used to align *colour separations.*

reproduction computer A plastic disc with a rotating scale, used to calculate new reproduction sizes (in inches or centimetres) when artwork is enlarged or reduced by a given percentage.

resident memory The permanent memory that forms part of the computer. The resident memory is of two kinds, *read-only* and *random-access.*

resolution *See:* printer resolution; screen resolution.

reversed-out *See:* reversed type.

reversed type White type on a black background, as opposed to the more usual black type on a white background.

RGB A system of specifying colours on *VDUs* according to the percentage output of each of the three electron guns.

RIP *See:* raster image processor.

RISC Reduced Instruction Set Computing. An advanced standard for microprocessor chips used in *personal computers.* They have an advantage over *CISC* chips in that they are less expensive and far more efficient.

rivers White spaces running vertically through a passage of text. They occur when the *word spacing* is too great in relation to the *line spacing.*

ROM *See:* read-only memory.

rub-down lettering *See:* dry-transfer lettering.

S

sans serif Refers to typefaces without *serifs.*

saturation The perceived purity of a colour. A saturated colour is given by a narrow range of wavelengths of light, whereas an unsaturated colour has various other wavelengths mixed in with the *dominant wavelength.* This is the equivalent of adding white.

scanner A device capable of 'reading' black and white printed images and converting them into *binary* data that can be processed by a computer.

Scrapbook (Macintosh) A *desk accessory* that allows you to store useful items (logos, letterheads, diagrams etc.) and paste them into any *document* you are working on.

screen fonts *Fonts* exclusively for use on screen, or to represent printer fonts on screen. *See also:* printer fonts.

screen printing A printing process in which the image is photographed through a screen to break it up into tiny dots. The dots vary in size, becoming smaller in light areas and larger in dark areas, but all are so small that the overall appearance is of smooth tones.

screen refresh rate *See:* refresh rate.

screen resolution The number of *pixels* that can display horizontally and vertically. This varies according to the type of screen being used. May sometimes be described as the number of horizontal lines that the screen can accommodate. The lines may be interlaced (less sharp) or non-interlaced (sharper); this definition usually applies to television screens.

screening The process of photographing an image through a *halftone* screen to break it into a pattern of dots. This allows *continuous tone* images to be reproduced on a printing press using *process colours.* *Tints* of both *spot colours* and process colours can be obtained in the same way.

scrolling Moving the contents of a *file* so that a new section is visible on the screen or in a *window.*

SCSI An abbreviation for Small Computer System Interface. This is a standard interface for high-speed communication with *peripherals.*

search and replace The process of finding a specified string of *characters* wherever it occurs in a file and replacing it with another specified string. The better word-processing programs offer this facility.

secondary colour *See:* complementary colour.

serif Serifs are small finishing marks at the ends of the strokes making up a *character.*

set solid The term arose in relation to metal

type. When lines of type are butted to-gether without any *leading*, the type is said to be 'set solid'. The same term is sometimes used to describe *digital type* where the *linefeed* is the same as the *point size*.

set width With metal type, the width of the *type body* varies from one *character* to an-other. Character widths are specified by the *unit system* of measurement. The *em* is divided into units and each character is assigned a unit value, or set width. The concept of set width is also used in relation to *digital type*, even though there is no physical type body.

SGML An abbreviation for Standard Gen-eralised Mark-up Language. This is a complex *generic coding* scheme that has been adopted by the International Or-ganisation for Standardisation and the British Standards Institution.

ShareWare Public domain software, dis-tributed free or for a nominal fee.

show-through Dark shadows on the page, caused by type on the other side of the paper showing through. The greater the *opacity* of the paper, the less the show-through will be. The effects are mini-mised when the type areas on the two sides of each page are accurately backed-up.

signature A section of a book, usually con-sisting of 8 or 16 pages. The first page of each section usually carries a small let-ter or number to ensure that the sections are bound together in the correct se-quence.

small caps A smaller size of capital letters, often used when words embedded in a text passage need to be set in capitals. Small capitals help to preserve an even texture.

softcopy Data in electronic form.

software The *programs* used to drive a com-puter.

spot colour A colour printed on a printing press with a pre-mixed ink.

spread *See*: double-page spread.

spreadsheet A program that allows nu-merical data to be entered in rows and columns and then manipulated. A mod-elling tool much used for projections in business.

s/s An abbreviation used to indicate that a piece of *artwork* should be reproduced the same size.

stand-alone A computer that is not part of a *network*.

startup disc A disc that contains the *program files* necessary to start the computer working. With Macintosh computers, a startup disc must have the *systems folder* on it.

storyboard A method of planning a slide/OHP presentation or video. Sketches of the images are accompanied by notes on the spoken words that go with them.

subscript A small character set below the *baseline*. Much used in chemistry.

superscript A small character set above the *baseline*. Much used in mathematics, and in text to indicate the presence of a note or bibliographical reference.

superslide A square slide format which fits the standard 35mm slide projector, but cannot be made using standard 35mm film.

symmetric layout A page layout that has a central axis. Headings are usually cen-tred and the text *justified*.

System 7 One of the more advanced up-grades of system software for the Macintosh, incorporating many operat-ing enhancements.

systems folder (Macintosh and Power PC) A *folder* that contains the systems *pro-grams* necessary for the operation of a Macintosh computer.

T

terminal A keyboard and/or screen giving access to a *multi-user* computer system.

tiling Printing a large image as a number of smaller segments or 'tiles'. For example, an A2 image could be created on a *laser-printer* by dividing it into four A4 tiles.

tint A *spot colour* or *process colour* that has been screened to produce a lighter shade. *See also*: screening.

tonal value The *lightness* or darkness of a colour.

tools (Macintosh) Options available in 'paint', 'draw' and page make-up pro-grams. Typical tools include brushes and pens of different widths, a spray-paint facility, rules of different widths, an eraser, and so on. Tools are usually represented by *icons*.

tracking The reduction of the space between letters by the same amount for every letter combination. *See also*: kerning.

trim marks Marks used to indicate final page size. For example, if you are preparing a publication whose final page size will be smaller than A4, your laserprinted A4 pages will need trim marks. These are placed one in each corner, outside the final page area.

TrueType™ Scalable fonts from one outline. This means that one set of metrics is used to produce a variety of *character* sizes. This is more efficient and less RAM memory is used than with non-scalable fonts.

type body *See*: body size.

type family The complete range of *type styles* available within a *typeface*.

type size *See*: point size.

type style A variant of a *typeface*, e.g. bold, italic, condensed.

type weight Most *typefaces* are available in several different 'weights' or stroke thicknesses. A 'medium' or 'light' weight is usually used for continuous text, while 'bold' is useful for emphasis. Terms describing type weights are relative. 'Medium' in one typeface may be the visual equivalent of 'bold' in another.

typeface A set of letters, numerals, punctuation marks etc. with the same design characteristics.

typescale A metal or plastic device used to determine the *baseline-to-baseline measurement* between lines of type, or to find out how much space will be occupied by a given number of lines with a particular *linefeed*. Some typescales resemble ordinary rulers, but are marked in units of, say, 9, 10, 11 and 12 points; others are wider and slatted, and may allow you to measure as many as 15 different linefeeds.

U

unit system A relative system of measurement used to specify *set widths* of characters, *letter spacing*, and sometimes *word spacing*.

The width of the *em* is divided vertically into a fixed number of units. (With metal type there are usually 18 units to the em, but the current industry standard for *laser typesetters* is 54 units to the em.) The actual width of the unit depends on the *point size* of the type: in an 18-unit system, the unit would be 1 point wide with 18pt type and half a point wide with 9pt type.

Each character is then assigned a width of so many units, including a small amount of space on either side to separate it from its neighbours. This is 'standard' letter spacing. In an 18-unit system, 'M' might have a width of 18 units, 'h' 10 units, and 'i' 5 units.

UNIX A *multi-user*, multi-tasking operating system that allows several people to use the same computer at the same time.

uppercase letters Another way of describing capital letters. *See also*: lowercase letters.

UserWare *Software* that is available to all for a nominal fee. *See also shareware*.

V

VDU An abbreviation for 'visual display unit'.

vector-mapping The storage of an image in terms of vectors and coordinates.

vertical justification The adjustment of line spacing to make a block of text fit within a designated area.

visual acuity The resolving power of the human eye.

W

widow The final line of a paragraph, isolated at the top of the next column or page.

WIMP An abbreviation for a system using *windows, icons*, a *mouse*, and *pull-down menus*.

Winchester An alternative name, now little used, for a *hard disc*.

window In some computer systems (such as Macintosh), documents are viewed through 'windows' on the *desktop*. Windows can be moved around or changed in size. Some *programs* allow you to have several windows open at once on the desktop. This is ideal for *cut-and-paste* operations.

word spacing The space between words. Usually an *en*, or one-third of an *em*.

word wrap The automatic carry-over of text to the next line when the *measure* is full.

WYSIWYG An abbreviation for 'what you see is what you get', meaning that, for example, if you specify bold type you will see bold type on the screen as well as on the final printout. Neither the resolution nor the measurements of the screen image will match the printed image exactly.

X

x-height The height of the *lowercase* letter 'x', measured from the *baseline* to the *mean line*. The x-height is used as a measure of the size of the lowercase letters in a given *typeface* and size, excluding the *ascenders* and *descenders*.

xerography An electrostatic copying process. The original is exposed onto a metal drum which becomes electrostatically charged in areas where dark lines are present. The charge attracts powdered ink or 'toner', which is then transferred to paper and fused to it by heat.

Z

zoom A facility that allows the entire page to be viewed at a reduced size, or small portions to be viewed at enlarged sizes.

FURTHER READING AND OTHER NOTES

Writing

Baron DN *Units, symbols and abbreviations: a guide for medical and scientific editors and authors* (5th edn). London: Royal Society of Medicine Press 1994. Essential reading for the scientific writer. Contains nearly all the SI units and useful notes on reference methods and proof correction marks.

Carey GV *Mind the stop* (revised edn). Harmondsworth: Penguin 1958. The do's and don'ts of punctuation, clearly explained.

Fowler HW (revised by Sir Ernest Gowers) *A dictionary of modern English usage* (2nd edn). Oxford: Oxford University Press 1965.

Gowers E (revised by S Greenbaum and J Whitcut) *The complete plain words* (3rd edn). London: Her Majesty's Stationery Office 1986. The classic guide to the use of English. Very readable.

Hall GM (ed) *How to write a paper*. London: BMJ Publishing Group 1994.

Kirkman J *Full marks* (2nd edn). Marlborough: Ramsbury Books 1993. Obtainable from bookshops, price £5.95 (pbk), or from Ramsbury Books, P0 Box 106, Marlborough, Wiltshire, SN8 2RU. Add 61p for postage in UK, £1.10 elsewhere in Europe, £2.51 outside Europe. Advice on punctuation for scientific and technical writing.

Kirkman J *Guidelines for giving effective presentations*. Marlborough: Ramsbury Books 1994. Obtainable from bookshops, price £7.95 (pbk), or from Ramsbury Books, P0 Box 106, Marlborough, Wiltshire, SN8 2RU. Add 61p for postage in UK, £1.18 elsewhere in Europe, £2.51 outside Europe.

O'Connor M *Writing successfully in science*. London: Chapman & Hall 1991. Pbk £8.95, hbk £25.00.

Partridge E *Usage and abusage* (revised edn). London: Hamish Hamilton 1965. An alphabetical survey of words and constructions that are frequently misused.

Strunk W Jr and White EB *The elements of style* (3rd edn). New York: Macmillan; London: Collier Macmillan 1979. A concise guide to style in written English.

Turk C and Kirkman J *Effective writing: improving scientific, technical and business communication*. London: E & F N Spon 1982. One of the best books of its kind.

House style

Butcher J *Copy editing: the Cambridge handbook* (2nd edn). Cambridge: Cambridge University Press 1982. Perhaps the classic among English style manuals.

Hart H *Hart's rules for compositors and readers at the University Press Oxford* (39th edn). London: Oxford University Press 1983. A concise reference book on house style.

University of Chicago Press *The Chicago manual of style for authors, editors and copywriters* (14th edn). Chicago: University of Chicago Press 1993. Gives exhaustive coverage of every aspect of editing and book production. An invaluable reference book

Electronic manuscripts

Quorum Technical Services *Typesetting for micro users: a beginner's guide to improved text presentation*. Cheltenham: Quorum Technical Services Ltd 1985. A step-by-step guide to the use of generic coding in electronic manuscripts. Invaluable for those who wish to prepare manuscripts using a word-processing system and then send the discs to a professional typesetter.

University of Chicago Press *Chicago guide to preparing electronic manuscripts*. Chicago:

University of Chicago Press 1987. A guide for both authors and publishers. It discusses the division of labour between author and publisher, and explains how the electronic manuscript should be keyboarded and generically coded.

Dorner J *Writing on disc: an A-Z handbook of terms, tips and techniques for authors and publishers*. John Taylor Book Ventures 1992. Available by mail order from Spa Books, telephone 0462 482812.

Desktop publishing

Felici J and Nace T *Desktop publishing skills: a primer for typesetting with computers and laser printers*. Wokingham: Addison-Wesley 1987. Contains much helpful information on systems and equipment, and how to select them. The typographic features offered by electronic typesetting systems are clearly explained, and there are chapters on typeface selection and page layout.

Luna P *Understanding type for desktop publishing*. London: Blueprint 1992. An excellent guide for those who want to know more about typefaces.

Miles J *Design for desktop publishing: a guide to layout and typography on the personal computer*. London: Gordon Fraser Gallery Ltd 1987. Concerned mainly with design principles rather than computing. Profusely illustrated.

Parker RC *The Aldus guide to basic design*. Seattle, Washington: Aldus Corporation 1987. This is an excellent pocket-size guide, full of helpful illustrations and ideas for layout, from books to newspapers. Highly recommended.

Wilson-Davies K, St John Bate J and Barnard M *Desktop publishing*. London: Blueprint Publishing Ltd 1987. Written for publishers, this book explains the technology of desktop publishing and compares the most popular systems.

Legibility

Reynolds L Legibility studies: their relevance to present-day documentation

methods. *Journal of Documentation* 1979 **35** (4) 307-340. A survey of the results of research on legibility, including work carried out since Spencer's 'The visible word' was published.

Spencer H *The visible word*. London: Lund Humphries 1969. The classic survey of legibility research, beautifully illustrated. Out of print, but obtainable through libraries.

Tinker M *Legibility of print*. Ames, Iowa: Iowa State University Press 1963. Tinker devoted many years to the study of legibility, covering such topics as typeface, type size, line length, line spacing, and so on. This is a summary of his findings. Out of print, but obtainable through libraries.

Typography and layout

Craig J *Designing with type* (revised edn). New York: Watson-Guptill; London: Pitman 1980. A practical guide, pitched at a level suitable for those with little previous knowledge of typography.

Hartley J *Designing instructional text*. London: Kogan Page 1978. Practical recommendations for the design of textbooks and teaching materials, backed up by summaries of relevant research results.

McLean R *The Thames and Hudson manual of typography*. London: Thames and Hudson 1980. A thorough coverage of the principles and techniques of typographic design. Historical detail is given where appropriate.

Colour

Binns B *Designing with two colours*. New York: Watson Guptill 1991. Gives examples of ways of using a second colour in text and illustrations.

Osborne R *Lights and pigments: colour principles for artists*. London: John Murray 1980. A very readable introduction to colour perception, colour mixing, colour measurement and colour reproduction (both additive and subtractive).

White JV *Colour for the electronic age*. New York: Watson Guptill; Oxford: Phaidon

1990. Demonstrates the importance of using colour meaningfully in text and illustration and includes some wonderful examples of colour badly used.

Tables

Ehrenberg ASC *Data reduction: analysing and interpreting statistical data*. London: John Wiley 1975. Contains useful advice on the construction of tables.

Wright P and Fox K *Presenting information in tables. Applied Ergonomics* 1970 **1** 134-242. Describes original research on the design of tables.

Graphs, charts and diagrams

Cleveland WS *The elements of graphing data*. Monterey, California: Wadsworth Advanced Books and Software 1985. A study of the methods and principles of graph construction. Recommendations are backed up by the results of research on the perception of graphs.

Lockwood A *Diagrams: a visual survey of graphs, maps, charts and diagrams*. London: Studio Vista 1969. Very little text, but superbly illustrated.

Tufte E *The visual display of quantitative information*. Cheshire, Connecticut: Graphics Press 1983. A survey of methods of presenting quantitative data, with many wonderful examples. The concepts of 'data ink' and 'chart junk' are explained. Obtainable from Graphics Press, PO Box 430, Cheshire, Connecticut 06410, USA, price $36 post-paid (hbk).

Tufte E *Envisioning information*. Cheshire, Connecticut: Graphics Press 1990. A visual feast, not to be missed by anyone interested in graphs and charts. Obtainable from Graphics Press, PO Box 430, Cheshire, Connecticut 06410, USA, price $48 post-paid (hbk).

Wright P *Presenting technical information: a survey of research findings. Instructional Science* 1977 **6** 93-134. A thorough and very useful survey by one of the leading researchers in this area.

Copyright

Cavendish JM and Pool K *Handbook of copyright in British publishing practice*. London: Cassell 1993. Available from booksellers or the Society of Authors, price £35 (hbk). Very clear and comprehensive, covering photocopying, use of illustrations, commissioning work and working for an employer, what to look out for when signing agreements plus many other aspects of the subject.

British Standards

British Standards can be obtained from:

The British Standards Institution
2 Park Street
London W1A 2B
Telephone 071 629 9000

Specification for numbering of divisions and subdivisions in written documents (point-numbering). BS 5848 : 1980

Guide to presentatin of tables and graphs. BS 7581 : 1992

Letter symbols, signs and abbreviations. BS 1991 : 1976

Specification for SI units and recommendations for the use of their multiples and of certain other units BS 5555 : 1993

Specification for abbreviation of title words and titles of publications. BS 4148 : 1985

Recommendation for references to published materials. BS 1629 : 1989

Recommendations for citing and referencing published material. BS 5605 : 1990

Recommendations for preparing indexes to books, peridoicals and other documents. BS 3700 : 1988

Copy preparation and proof correction. Recommendations for preparation of typescript copy for printing. BS 5261 : Part 1 : 1975

Copy preparation and proof correction. Specification for typographic requirements, marks for copy preparation and proof correction, proofing procedure. BS 5261 : Part 2 : 1976

Copy preparation and proof correction. Marks for copy preparation and proof correction. [Extracted from BS 5261 : Part 2 : 1976] BS 5261C : 1976

Copy preparation and proof correction. Specification for marks for mathematical copy preparation and mathematical proof correction and their uses. BS 5261 : Part 3 : 1989

Sizes of paper and board. Specification for A and B series of trimmed sizes of writing paper and certain classes of printed matters. BS 4000 : Part 1 : 1990

Sizes of paper and board. Specification for untrimmed sizes. BS 4000 : Part 2 : 1983

Notes

Helmono, a monospaced font for better projection, is available from:

Doig Simmonds
23 Bellevue Road
Ealing
London W13 8DF

The Society of Authors gives free advice to members on all aspects of writing and publishing, including finding illustrators. The Society is particularly helpful when contracts with publishers are being considered.

The Society of Authors
84 Drayton Gardens
London SW10 9SB
Telephone 071 373 6642
Fax 071 373 5768

Technical leaflets on photographic materials for slides and overhead transparencies are available from:

Kodak Ltd
PO Box 66
Kodak House
Station Road
Hemel Hempstead
Hertfordshire HP1 1UJ

Leaflet No. E 30 *Storage and care of Kodak film and papers before and after processing.* Useful advice on the care of colour slides in various climatic areas.

Leaflet No. E 943 (H) *Kodak Ektachrome and overhead materials.* Deals with materials for the overhead projector.

INDEX